CONTENTS

Introduction 8

    What you will learn in this book...9

Chapter 1: Introduction to Keto Veganism 10

    What is the Ketogenic Diet?... 10

    The Science Behind Ketosis and How it Aids in Weight Loss Management 12

    How The Keto Ketogenic Diet and Vegan Diets Differ 14

    What is the Keto Vegan Diet?.. 14

    Benefits of Keto Vegan Diet 16

    How to Get Started with the Keto Vegan Diet 17

Chapter 2: What to Eat on Keto Vegan Diet..................................... 19

    Foods That Should be Avoided on the Keto Vegan Diet 19

    Foods That You Can Eat on the Keto Vegan Diet................................... 19

    Common Mistakes People Make on the Keto Vegan Diet and How to Avoid Them
    20

Chapter 3: Meal Plan, Preparation and Storage 22

    21-Day Keto Vegan Meal Plan.. 22

    Keto Vegan Shopping List... 25

    Preparing and Storing Food on the Keto Vegan Diet............................ 26

Chapter 4: Sauces and Condiments Recipes 27

    Keto Salsa Verde 27

    Chimichurri.. 28

    Keto Vegan Raw Cashew Cheese Sauce 28

Spicy Avocado Mayonnaise..29

Green Coconut Butter 30

Spiced Almond Butter...30

Keto Strawberry Jam..31

Chocolate Coconut Butter..31

Orange Dill Butter 32

Keto Caramel Sauce 32

Pecan Butter 33

Keto Vegan Ranch Dressing...33

Cauliflower Hummus 34

Cauliflower Cream..34

Eggplant Dip 35

Chapter 5: Breakfast Recipes...36

Cauliflower Berry Breakfast Bowl 36

No - Fuss Breakfast Cereal 37

Easy Breakfast Bagels 38

Cranberry Breakfast Bars..39

Pumpkin Spice Pancakes 40

Lemon Pancakes 41

Keto Vegan Vanilla French Toast..42

Cashew Yogurt Bowl 42

Cinnamon Coconut Porridge 43

Zucchini Breakfast Bars 43

Overnight Coconut Pumpkin Porridge...44

Cheesy Scrambled Tofu..45

Chocolate Waffles...46

Macadamia Nut Bars..47

Spaghetti Squash Hashbrowns...48

Blueberry Scones..49

Chocolate Zucchini Pancakes...50

Avocado Breakfast Bowl..51

4 Seed Keto Vegan Bread...52

Cashew Coconut Breakfast Bars..52

Chapter 6: Lunch Recipes 53

Quick and Easy Cucumber Tomato Salad...53

Oven Baked Spicy Cauliflower Wings...54

Spicy Cucumber Salad..55

Grilled Tofu Skewers...56

Creamy Tomato Soup..57

Avocado Zucchini Noodles..58

Creamy Pumpkin Soup..58

Lime Coconut Cauliflower Rice...59

Sautéed Jackfruit Cauliflower Bowl...60

Tuna Imitation Salad...61

Lettuce Salad Bowls...62

Keto Vegan Empanadas..63

Avocado Fries...64

Sautéed Squash Kale Bowl 65

Avocado Cauliflower Salad 65

Mushroom Cauliflower Soup 66

Zucchini Veggie Wraps 67

Cauliflower Cabbage Wraps 68

Zucchini Green Bean Salad...69

Quick and Easy Cauliflower Pizza Bites 70

Chapter 7: Dinner Recipes...71

Cauliflower Steaks...72

Veggie Walnut Soup 73

Roasted Red Pepper Soup 74

Zucchini Spinach Ravioli..75

Keto Vegan Shepherd's Pie 76

Green Soup 78

Portobello Mushroom Tacos with Guacamole 79

Roasted Mushroom Burgers 80

Roasted Radishes...81

Roasted Pepper Zoodles 82

Creamy Curry Zucchini Noodles 83

Creamy Spinach Shirataki 84

Tempeh Broccoli Stir Fry Dinner..85

Sautéed Brussel Sprouts Dish..86

Cauliflower Pizza Crust with Veggie Toppings 87

Tofu Tomato Stir Fry.. 88

Walnut Zucchini Chili 89

Roasted Veggies on Broccoli Rice 90

Keto Vegan Thai Curry.. 91

Falafel with Tahini Sauce.. 92

Chapter 8: Dessert and Snacks Recipes... 93

Baked Zucchini Chips.. 93

Gluten-Free Nut-Free Red Velvet Cupcakes 94

5-Ingredient Ice-cream.. 95

Peanut Butter Cups.. 96

Chocolate Avocado Mousse 97

Spiced Kale Chips... 98

Coconut Fat Cups... 99

Almond Coconut Fat Cups 100

Candied Toasted Cashew Nuts 101

Almond Cookies 102

Coconut Protein Crackers... 103

Raw Strawberry Crumble... 104

Peanut Butter Energy Bars 105

Lemon Squares.. 106

Apple Cider Donuts.. 107

Chapter 9: Smoothies and Other Beverage Recipes 108

Matcha Spinach Smoothie 108

Protein-Packed Blueberry Smoothie 109

Chocolate Avocado Smoothie... 109

Mint Cauliflower Smoothie 110

Strawberry Protein Smoothie... 110

Turmeric Avocado Smoothie 111

Raspberry Avocado Smoothie 111

Vanilla Coconut Smoothie 112

Cleansing Green Spinach Juice.. 112

Lime Kale Juice 113

Berry Spinach Juice.. 113

Keto Vegan Hot Chocolate.. 114

Iced Coffee Latte.. 115

Keto Vegan Eggnog 116

Creamy Golden Milk 116

Introduction

Veganism is a vegetarian diet that excludes the use of products derived from animals including but not limited to their meat, dairy products, and eggs. Veganism is a popular diet, and this is due in part to its many health-related benefits, which include:

- Reducing the risk of developing cardiovascular diseases such as heart disease, stroke and high blood pressure. Veganism promotes the consumption of fruits, vegetables, whole grains, nuts and legumes, all of which provide valuable nutrition that improves cardiovascular function and therefore, lowers the risk of developing cardiovascular diseases.
- Providing valuable nutrition that is often deficit in normal eating routines. We live in a fast-paced world and often our diet, and therefore overall health, suffer as a result. Veganism allows you to be more conscious of what you eat and to obtain higher amounts of nutrients like fiber, potassium, magnesium, vitamin A, vitamin C, vitamin D and antioxidants that are often missing in "convenient" products that are on store shelves and available at fast-food restaurants.
- Providing protection against certain cancers. The same products on store shelves and in fast-food restaurants that claim to be convenient are often detrimental to your health in the long run as they introduce unsafe products to the diet. Poor diet practices often lead to cancer development. Therefore, the healthier consumption of food products on the vegan diet significantly lowers the risk of developing certain cancers, namely breast, prostate and colon cancer.
- Decreasing inflammation throughout the body. Raw foods are often consumed on a vegan diet. In fact, there is a type of veganism whereby the practitioner consumes only raw food products. Raw foods are rich in antioxidants and probiotics which helps decrease chronic inflammation, which is an overreaction of the immune system. This can also decrease the symptoms of rheumatoid arthritis which include swelling, joint pain and morning sickness.

These are only a few of the many health benefits gained by practicing veganism. Others include improved kidney function, lowered blood sugar levels, and decreased risk of developing type 2 diabetes. The benefits of practicing veganism are not just dietary or health-related though. There are many lifestyle benefits as well.

There is a saying that goes, "If you stand for nothing then you will fall for anything." There is a lot that is wrong in this world and many of these injustices are perpetrated in the name of helping humanity and advancing our way of life. One of the greatest injustices that has going on throughout the ages is the killing, torture, and harm of animals to sustain human life. Animals should not have to suffer so that we can eat or be protected from the elements when there are alternative sources for food, clothing, shelter and more that are naturally given. Animals should not suffer so that we can purchase clothing, wear makeup, or use sanitary products. Animals should not be treated cruelly or die simply because we want to live a certain lifestyle. Especially if living that lifestyle can be attained by much safer, greener, and animal cruelty-free means.

In the same regard, deforestation should not be rampant, the use of global resources should not be strained and the protection of the environment should be paramount. However, that is not the way it is. Instead, deforestation is a growing problem, the strain on global resources is becoming heavier, and the environment continues to suffer. This happens all in the name of farming and the upkeep of livestock and other animals.

Going vegan can completely change the world and the way it operates. Going vegan does not just describe a diet. It describes a lifestyle. It goes way past what we choose to eat and extends to how we live. Being a vegan means that you completely stop supporting practices that exploit animals for profit or gain. Just as human beings have the right to live freely and happily, these rights should be extended to our animal counterparts. They are an essential part of the circle of life and killing or harming them will ultimately harm humanity and the Earth itself.

This book is about showing you what it means to be vegan as well as how you can lose weight naturally and quickly from a popular diet that seems to go against everything a vegan lifestyle entails. This diet is called the ketogenic diet. The ketogenic diet is a high-fat diet that promotes the reduction of carbohydrates so that the body can use energy in a more efficient and cleaner way. Even though this is a high-fat diet, it is very effective at helping the practitioner lose weight safely and naturally.

Unfortunately, the "gurus" of the ketogenic diet often promote the consumption of animals and their byproducts to achieve the benefits that this diet offers. The good news is that you as a vegan can still hold your ideals for practicing a vegan lifestyle while reaping the benefits of the ketogenic diet. This book was created to show you how you can do this without ever harming or consuming animals and their byproducts.

What you will learn in this book

- The difference between the ketogenic diet and the vegan diet
- What is the ketogenic vegan diet
- The benefits of practicing the keto vegan diet
- What it means to live a keto vegan lifestyle
- The steps you can take before starting such a lifestyle
- How you can lose weight naturally with the keto vegan diet
- The foods to eat and to avoid on the ketogenic vegan diet
- A 21-day meal plan
- How to prepare and store food on the keto vegan diet
- How to grocery shop to suit your keto vegan lifestyle, including a comprehensive shopping list
- Recipes for breakfast, lunch, dinner, smoothies, desserts and more

In addition to being a comprehensive guidebook for the transition into a keto vegan lifestyle, this book provides tasty recipes that have a powerful effect on your body as it relates to weight loss and improving overall health. Eating healthy does not translate into boring, tasteless food. You can lose weight, improve your cardiovascular health, improve your kidney function and the host of many other health-related benefits of veganism while still treating your taste buds to something good and delicious with every single meal. In the upcoming pages, you will find over 100 recipes for breakfast, lunch, dinner, dessert, snacks and more that will delight your taste buds, help you lose weight, improve your mental function, help elevate your mood and more!

Thank you for downloading this book. My hope is that you gain extreme value with every word that you read so that you can live a healthier and happier life while upholding ideals that will benefit not only the planet and animals but future generations as well.

Chapter 1: Introduction to Keto Veganism

With a surface glance, the ketogenic diet, a diet which thrives off of receiving higher amounts of fat and protein from mainly animal-based products and the vegan diet, which is one that strictly forbids the use of any animal-based products, seem to have nothing in common. But things are hardly ever as they seem from first glance. Take a deeper look and you will see how combining these two diets can completely change your life and improve your health holistically.

What is the Ketogenic Diet?

The human body needs fuel to perform. This fuel often comes in the form of carbohydrates. The simplest form of carbohydrate is called sugar. The cycle of getting energy from sugar starts with the consumption of food that contains sugar. This causes a spike in insulin levels and the liver turns sugar into fat. As the sugar enters the bloodstream, it causes blood pressure to rise. In addition, the consumption of sugar has an effect similar to heroin on the brain. It makes the consumer feel happy because the brain produces high levels of the hormone called dopamine in response to its presence.

As a result, the person experiences high levels of energy, elevated mood, and a feeling similar to a drug user's high. This effect does not last long. Insulin levels begin to rapidly fall and so the person feels very tired as their energy levels decrease. Their mood also changes as dopamine levels begin to fall.

In response, the body demands more sugar which starts a chronic cycle of addiction and dependency on sugar. Sugar is eight times more addictive than cocaine and having a sweet tooth may be more dangerous than you realize. Most people do not even realize that they are addicted to sugar but there are signs that clearly indicate a sugar addiction and they include:

- Craving comfort food in response to both high and low times in your life.
- Craving sweet foods and beverages.
- Rewarding accomplishments with sugary food.
- Experiencing physical withdrawal symptoms when going without sugary foods for even a short amount of time.
- Trying to stay away from sugary foods unsuccessfully
- Binge eating sugary foods.

The Consequences of Sugar Addiction

Sugar has many negative effects on the body. They include:

- Causing the growth of bacteria in the mouth which can lead to bad breath and cavities.
- Increasing the risk of developing cardiovascular diseases. This is caused by the extra insulin that excessive sugar intake produces. This extra insulin causes the walls of blood vessels to grow faster than normal and become rigid. The resulting tautness of the blood vessels, narrow space available for blood to travel. This places extra stress on the heart, which can lead to cardiovascular diseases such as heart attack and stroke.
- Increasing the risk of developing type 2 diabetes. Insulin is produced by the pancreas, which works overtime when excessive sugar is introduced into the body. This can lead to the development of type 2 diabetes.
- Increasing the risk of kidney damage. The kidneys filter blood sugar and the extra work resulting from the excessive intake of sugar can cause damage.
- Causing erectile dysfunction in men. The function of the cardiovascular system becomes impaired due to excessive insulin levels. This causes interruptions in the blood supplied to the groin, which causes impaired sexual function.

● Causing inflammation, which can cause joint pain and increase the risk of developing rheumatoid arthritis. Inflammation also causes the skin to age faster because it breaks down proteins in the skin and causes the creation of harmful molecules called Advanced Glycation End-products (AGEs). These molecules cause the skin to lose its elasticity and therefore, to form wrinkles.

These are only a few of the negative effects that excessive intake of sugar can cause. These negative consequences extend to sugar's contribution to excessive weight gain and obesity.

Obesity and its Health Implications

Obesity is a disease that occurs when a person carries excessive body weight or body fat which has adverse effects on their health.

Unfortunately, this is a far-reaching disease. More than 90 million Americans were affected by obesity between the years 2015 and 2016 in the US. It was estimated that 1 in 5 adults were morbidly obese in the United States in 2017. These are truly staggering figures because no one is born obese or has to become obese! Obesity is often a consequence of lifestyle and diet choices, both of which are normally within a person's control.

Obesity is determined by the use of body mass index also known as BMI. BMI is an assessment of whether or not a person carries the appropriate amount of weight for their age and height. A BMI of 30 and over means that a person is obese. A BMI between 25 and 29.9 indicates that a person is carrying excess weight but is not yet obese. A BMI between 18.5 and 24.9 indicates that a person carries a healthy weight. A BMI that is below 18.5 means that a person is underweight and needs to gain weight.

The implications of obesity are far-reaching. This disease does not occur in isolation. It increases the risk of developing many other health complications such as:

● Cardiovascular disease. This occurs because obesity places a strain on the cardiovascular system. It also causes a rise in blood pressure and cholesterol levels.
● Type 2 diabetes. Excessive weight gain has an adverse effect on the production of insulin and blood sugar levels, which can increase the risk of developing insulin resistance and therefore, type 2 diabetes.
● Sleep apnea. Sleep apnea occurs when a person stops breathing for a few seconds intermittently. Obesity increases the likelihood of developing this condition, which can lead to death.
● Certain cancers. Fat deposits are often seen as a foreign entity by the body and as such, the immune system attacks the body in an effort to get rid of them. This causes the deformation of cells and tissues and produces an environment conducive to the development of cancer cells. As a result, certain cancers such as ovarian, colon, breast, rectum, liver, pancreas, prostate and kidney have been linked to obesity.
● Osteoarthritis. Excessive weight gain places stress on the joints, which increases inflammation and therefore, the risk of developing this condition.
● Digestive issues. A person who is overweight is more likely to develop digestive issues such as problems with liver function, gallbladder disease, and heartburn to name a few.

These are only a few of the negative health implications that are linked to obesity. Luckily, these diseases and obesity can be prevented and reversed by changing your diet and not relying on carbohydrates as your body's primary source of energy and fuel. The ketogenic diet provides the body with an alternative source of energy that does not have these negative effects.

The ketogenic diet is a low-carb, high-fat and moderate protein diet that places the body in a metabolic state called ketosis. The ketogenic diet is one that entails a daily meal plan that consists of between 5 and 10% carbohydrates, 20 and 25% protein and 70 and 75% fat. On this diet, the average person will consume less than 50 grams of carbohydrates for the day. This forces the person's body to rely on an alternative source of energy rather than carbohydrates. This alternate source is body fat.

The Science Behind Ketosis and How it Aids in Weight Loss Management

The reason that the ketogenic diet is so efficient at not only causing weight loss but improving overall health is that it replaces carbohydrate intake with healthy fat intake. This shifts the body away from metabolizing carbohydrates and towards metabolizing fat in an effort to gain energy. Simply put, when you practice the ketogenic diet, your body no longer uses standard sugar to gain energy but instead burns body fat, which can lead to weight loss in addition to many more significant health benefits.

The ketogenic diet has been around for over 100 years and was initially developed in an effort to fight epilepsy. However, its many other health benefits and its efficiency at causing weight loss cannot be denied.

This diet causes weight loss through a process known as ketosis. Ketosis is a metabolic state that only occurs when foods that are rich in carbohydrates are restricted. This restriction forces the body to look for alternative fuel sources and it turns to fat for that source. Ketosis can occur naturally such as when a person is fasting, during pregnancy or during starvation. If you have ever skipped a meal or two or partook in strenuous exercise then you have likely undergone this process unknowingly. Practicing the ketogenic diet is a less extreme way of forcing the body to seek out alternative sources of energy.

The process is so named because the fat molecules transformed into an energy source are called ketones. Ketones are fat-derived energy molecules that are generated in the liver and flows through the bloodstream. When the term 'ketones' or 'ketone bodies' is used, it typically refers to three main types. The first two are called acetoacetate and beta-hydroxybutyrate. They are more abundant that the third type, which is called, acetone.

Ketones are always present in the blood, but their presence increases dramatically when there are conditions that force the body away from metabolizing carbohydrates. They are used by the major organs such as the brain, heart, and kidney. Ketosis and therefore, ketones are particularly important to the brain because the brain has no other way of deriving energy apart from the metabolism of carbohydrates and fats.

How Ketosis Occurs

Before the process of ketosis is activated, gluconeogenesis occurs. Gluconeogenesis is the process whereby used non-carbohydrate components like amino acids, which are the units from which proteins are made, produce energy. This process occurs when sugar intake is limited and glycogen, which is your body's storage of sugar is being used. As glycogen becomes depleted, gluconeogenesis increases and jumpstarts the fat burning process even though ketone production does not yet occur at this point.

The next stage occurs when glycogen is completed depleted. Gluconeogenesis completely takes over and ketones begin to be produced in low quantities. This is called the gluconeogenic phase. As the body does not get supplied with sufficient carbohydrates, ketosis occurs. This is characterized by a decrease in the use of non-carbohydrate components like amino acids to create energy and a complete shift to prioritizing the production of ketones.

Ketones are formed in the liver as fat cells get broken down in a process called ketogenesis. The first ketone that is produced is acetoacetate. Acetoacetate is then converted to beta-hydroxybutyrate, or BHB for short, and acetone. As your body adapts to gaining energy from ketosis, BHB becomes the most common ketone. When you full adapted to ketosis, ketones provide up to 50% of the body's base energy while catering to up to 70% of the brain's energy needs.

How Ketosis Causes Weight Loss

It might be difficult to understand how a diet can recommend the consumption of fat to lose weight while traditional diets preach the exact opposite. This might seem like madness to an outside observer. However, taking a closer look shows that the ketogenic diet promotes the burning of fat to form ketones, which leads to natural weight loss.

Also, because of the foods that are recommended for consumption are high in healthy fat and protein, the practitioner is left feeling fuller and more satisfied after every meal. This leads to not overeating and therefore, better weight reduction and metabolic health.

It also creates a reduction in appetite as well so that the person does not overeat by indiscriminately reaching for snacks during the day. Unfortunately, the most convenient snacks that are available happen to be those loaded in carbohydrates. Even if the person has healthy snack options but indulges is sweets too often, the results are often linked to weight gain. On the ketogenic diet, appetite is curbed to lessen the likelihood of reaching for unhealthy snacks or for snacking too much.

One of the most common problem areas that people experience when losing weight is the belly area. Belly fat consists of visceral fat, which is a type of fat that encases internal organs around the abdominal area. The build-up of this type of fat has been linked to the development of type 2 diabetes and heart disease. The ketogenic diet makes it possible to eliminate visceral fat because visceral fat production has been closely linked to the consumption of carbohydrates and refined sugars. Both of these are discouraged on the ketogenic diet which leads to a reduction of the development of this type of fat and therefore, weight loss in the abdominal area as well as all over the body.

Other Benefits of Ketosis

Ketosis is not just about fat burning. It has many serious and positive implications for your health and wellness. They include:

● The stimulation of mitochondrial production. Mitochondria are the part of body cells that generate the chemical energy needed to facilitate the cell's biochemical reactions. New mitochondria are synthesized in cells that used ketones as a fuel. This is especially prominent in brain cells. The formation of more mitochondria helps improve energy production and the overall health of cells.
● Ketones function similarly to an antioxidant. An antioxidant is a substance that removes potentially damaging oxidizing agents from forming in the body. Oxidation is a chemical process that occurs in cells and can produce free radicals, which are chemicals that damage cells. Vitamin C and E are popular antioxidants. Ketones produce less reactive oxygen and therefore, less free radicals than sugar and thus protects cells from damage.
● The protection and regeneration of nervous system cells. Ketosis aids in regenerating damaged nerve cells as well as preserving the function of aging nerve cells.
● Aids in preventing certain cancers. Most cancer cells cannot use ketones as fuel and therefore, die because they have nothing to facilitate their growth. This aids the immune system in removing them from the body.
● Aids in improving brain function. There have been promising studies on how the ketogenic diet and ketosis improve the brain function in people with autism, epilepsy, Alzheimer's disease, and Parkinson's disease, This can be attributed to the fact that the brain uses energy derived from ketones more effectively than it does with energy obtained from sugar. Ketosis also has an inhibitory effect on nerve cells, which makes the brain less excitable and therefore, more efficient in its function.
● Triggers the process of autophagy. Autophagy means "self-eating". It is the process whereby the body cleans out damaged cells and toxins in addition to regenerating new, healthier cells. Damaged cells and toxins accumulate over time if this process does not work efficiently. This causes several negative effects such as inducing dementia, increasing the risk of developing

certain cancers and accelerating aging. Consuming more fat on the ketogenic diet activates autophagy because your cells become more efficient at cleaning out old cells and regenerating new ones once it stops relying on carbohydrates to provide energy.

How The Keto Ketogenic Diet and Vegan Diets Differ

Both the ketogenic and vegan diets are great for their aid in weight loss management. However, individually, they take different approaches to doing so. The ketogenic diet, also known as the keto diet, emphasizes the consumption of fat and moderate protein. The most abundant sources of these are animal products like chicken, beef and fish, and animal-based products such as dairy products.

The vegan diet is completely different. It promotes the reduction of weight through plant-based eating and eliminates all food that comes from animal sources. The vegan diet is one that is rich in vegetables, fruits, and whole grains. Most vegans extend their diet into a lifestyle and do not use any products that involve the abuse, harm, or misuse of animals and their products. However, these two diets can be paired as quite the winning team for weight loss and improve overall health.

What is the Keto Vegan Diet?

While veganism is one of the healthiest diets because it promotes the consumption of naturally given animal-based products, the ketogenic diet is more effective for weight loss. Unfortunately, the ketogenic diet is not as environmentally-safe as the vegan diet. The keto vegan diet takes what is great about both of these diets and combines them into one diet that allows the practitioner to still eat healthy, clean and environmentally-safe while losing weight quickly and efficiently.

The keto vegan diet, also called the ketogenic vegan diet, is a high-fat, moderate protein and low carbohydrate diet that entails eating vegetable-based products only. This diet allows the practitioner to reap all the benefits of the ketogenic diet while still decreasing animal abuse and death, decreasing the carbon footprint and improving overall health.

This diet is so effective at allowing vegans to lose weight quickly and efficiently because it limits carbohydrate consumption to less than 50 grams per day. This is done through the consumption of low carb vegetables like cauliflower and broccoli and vegan-friendly protein sources like tofu, seeds, and nuts.

Unfortunately, many vegan-friendly favorites are filled with carbohydrates that defy the purpose of practicing the ketogenic diet. Some of these vegan-friendly favorites that are prohibited on the ketogenic diet include:
● Fruits such as bananas and apples.
● Natural sweeteners such as maple syrup and agave.
● Starchy vegetables such as potatoes and yams.
● Grains such as wheat, rice, and corn.
● Legumes like black beans and lentils.

All of these products are strictly prohibited on the ketogenic diet because they kick your body out of ketosis in order to metabolize the carbohydrates.

I will provide a comprehensive list of foods that are to be avoided and those to be consumed on the keto vegan diet, later on in this book. However, I will concentrate on how you can get enough fat to facilitate ketosis on the keto vegan diet in this section. Plant-based oils are a common replacement for animal fats in the keto vegan diet. They are commonly used in cooking, baking, making dressing, desserts, and a lot more. Here is a list of a few of these oils and how you can use them to make tasty dishes.

Olive oil. Olive oil is one of the healthiest oils that humans can consume because it is rich in monounsaturated fatty acids. It is great for stir-frying, sautéing, making dressings, sauces and condiments, baking and more. It can be used in both sweet and savory dishes. The benefits of this oil are far-reaching and extend past aiding in weight loss. It is also rich in antioxidants, has anti-inflammatory properties, helps improve cardiovascular health, and aids in reducing the development of type 2 diabetes.

Avocado oil. Avocado oil is rich in healthy monounsaturated fats and has a very high smoke point which is great for cooking, baking, and deep-frying. In addition to facilitating ketosis, this oil helps reduce cholesterol to improve heart health, enhances the absorption of fat-soluble nutrients, is rich in an antioxidant that helps improve eye health, and helps reduce the symptoms of arthritis.

Coconut oil. This oil is abundant in several types of fatty acids which is great for providing a fuel source for ketosis to occur. It is great for baking and cooking, for making desserts and as a primary ingredient in fat bombs. Recipes for fat bombs can be found in the dessert chapter. Coconut oil helps lower blood sugar levels, decreases the risk of developing type 2 diabetes, boosts good cholesterol, improves liver health and aids in digestion.

MCT oil. MCT stands for medium-chain triglycerides, which is a saturated fatty acid that skips the digestive process and goes straight to the liver where it is converted to ketones in the ketosis process. MCT oil is derived from coconut oil and palm oil and is a great addition to sauces, condiments, smoothies, fat bombs, salad dressings, and even hot drinks like coffee and tea. It is a potent energy booster.

Red palm oil. This can also be used as a vitamin supplement because it is a great source of both vitamin A and E. It enhances the flavor of several dishes because it has a mild buttery texture and carrot-like flavor. It is good to note that you should purchase red palm oil which is RSPO certified or a certified sustainable palm oil product as some of these products are made in environmentally unsafe ways.

Vegans are not limited to consuming plant-based oils to get the necessary intake of fat to facilitate ketosis. Avocados, nuts, seeds, and vegan dairy alternatives are also great sources of fat in addition to being packed with vitamins, minerals, and antioxidants.

Obtaining the necessary protein is also a concern on the keto vegan diet as animal products, which are the most common source of proteins is prohibited. Here are a few vegan-friendly protein sources that are safe to consume on the keto vegan diet:

- Tofu. Tofu is made from soybeans and is an excellent source of calcium and protein. It is a common substitute for meat, poultry, and fish because it can assume a texture that is similar and is great for absorbing flavor as it sucks up flavors from a marinade like a sponge.
- Tempeh. This is a fermented form of soy. It is firmer than tofu and has a grainy texture. It makes a great substitute for fish and ground beef.
- Seitan. This is a less common meat substitute that is made from wheat gluten, soy sauce, ginger, garlic, and seaweed. It is a great source of iron and protein. However, it must be noted that this protein substitute contains gluten and needs to be avoided if you have a sensitivity to gluten.
- Nuts and seeds. Examples of these include pumpkin seeds, pistachios, almonds, and flax seeds. They are naturally packed with protein. However, you should be careful with their consumption because they do contain some carb content. While peanuts are technically a legume, they are a low carb and high protein source and can be consumed in moderate quantities on the keto vegan diet.
- Protein powders. Protein powders are a great way of infusing your diet with protein. They are especially great additions to smoothies. Protein powders that are safe to be consumed on the keto vegan diet should be 100% plant-based protein and organic in nature. Some examples are soybean protein powder, mixed protein powder, or pea protein powder.

Vegan Alternatives to Eggs and Dairy

While the consumption of eggs and dairy are allowed on vegetarian diets, it is strictly prohibited on the vegan diet. Luckily, you can still get the nutrition that these two products provide with dairy replacements such as:

- Coconut cream for heavy cream
- Vegan butter or coconut oil for butter
- Vegan cheese, or nutritional yeast, for dairy-based cheeses
- Vegan soft cheese for cream cheese
- Vegan eggs and flax eggs for the use of eggs
- Nut-based yogurt such as cashew yogurt to replace yogurt and sour cream

Benefits of Keto Vegan Diet

We have discussed the major benefit of effective weight loss on the keto vegan diet. We have also discussed its contribution to lowering the risk of developing cardiovascular diseases and type 2 diabetes. Now, let's take a moment to go more in-depth in the other benefits of practicing this diet. Those benefits include:

- Having more energy throughout the day. On a carb-heavy diet, your body is constantly converting carbohydrates into sugar which elevates your blood sugar levels. While this results in an initial surge of energy, it soon becomes depleted and leaves you feeling less energetic and hungrier at fast intervals. This results in the chronic cycle of craving sugar and carbohydrates to get that energy back. Ketosis works differently from the metabolism of carbohydrates. Energy is maintained at consistent levels without spikes or drops. Also, there are no cravings for carbs on this diet, which leads to fewer feelings of hunger.
- Reducing the possibility of metabolic syndrome. Metabolic syndrome is a group of risk factors that increase your risk of developing heart disease and other related health problems such as type 2 diabetes and stroke. These risk factors include increased blood pressure, abdominal obesity, high blood sugar, high triglyceride (a type of fat) levels, and low HDL (good) cholesterol levels. You will be diagnosed with metabolic syndrome if you suffer 3 or more out of 5 of these risk factors. Practicing the keto vegan diet lowers your chances of developing these risk factors because it changes the way your body processes fat. Instead of being stored, fat is being used efficiently in the fat-converting process of ketosis.
- Improving sleep quality. Ketosis allows you to maintain steady energy levels throughout the day which makes it easier to fall asleep and stay asleep at night. Practicing the keto vegan diet also aids in the production of a chemical in the brain called adenosine, which aids in the regulation of the sleep cycle. This means that you are better able to fall asleep and wake up at the same time consistently every day. This helps with feeling more refreshed when awake and achieving Stage 4 REM sleep, which is the most restful and rejuvenating phase of sleep.
- Aids in making skin healthier and clearer. The consumption of carbohydrates results in inflammation which is one of the most common reasons that acne flare-ups occur. This occurs because insulin levels in the blood spike due to higher blood sugar levels. This results in higher oil production of oil in the skin, which leads to the clogging of follicles and breakouts. Consuming sugars and other carbohydrates also cause the skin to age faster because insulin causes the production of chemicals that erode the skin's elasticity, which causes wrinkles. On the other hand, consuming good fats prevents inflammation and does not induce the production of insulin. This results in fewer breakouts of pimples, blackheads, whiteheads, and other acne symptoms. The skin is also able to better maintain its elasticity. It also helps to soothe dry skin.
- Aids in the maintenance of a healthy digestive system. A healthy digestive system relies on the maintenance of a balanced environment where good bacteria can thrive, and nutrients are absorbed faster and more effectively. Certain bacteria in the digestive system help provide

your body with vitamins such as vitamins K and B12, which are essential in regulating your body's store of minerals like calcium. The metabolism of fat in the process of ketosis aids in maintaining a diverse and healthy environment for good bacteria to grow in the digestive system. On the other hand, the metabolism of carbohydrates can result in an imbalance of good and bad bacteria in the digestive system, which can have negative health implications.

● Aids in improving eyesight. Because the keto vegan diet is rich in good fats, it helps retinal cells in the eye maintain good health. This diet also prevents cell degeneration in that area. The symptoms of common eye problems such as cataracts and glaucoma have been shown to be reduced in persons who practice keto veganism.

● Improves mental health. Using fat as an energy source is far more efficient for the brain. Therefore, practicing keto veganism helps improve your focus and concentration as well as improve your critical thinking skills. Keto veganism also helps to clear up a protein called beta-amyloid. These proteins tend to stick together, which prevents fast and efficient flow of signals in the brain. This results in slowed thinking and reactions. By clearing this protein up, the keto vegan diet facilitates the faster and more efficient flow of signals in the brain as well as lowered risk of developing neurodegenerative diseases like Alzheimer's disease. It also helps reduce the symptoms of epilepsy. Epilepsy is a neurological disorder perpetuated by sudden recurring episodes of loss of consciousness, convulsions and sensory disturbances. These symptoms arise due to abnormal electrical activity the brains. The ketogenic diet is now famous for its weight loss benefits but it was actually initially created in the 1920s as a therapy to treat the symptoms of epilepsy. It aids by encouraging a mental environment that facilitates more normal electrical activity in the brain.

The keto vegan diet offers a wide array of health benefits because it combines high fat intake with low carb intake to boost nutrient absorption, to facilitate cleaner, faster internal processes and to improve the operation of mental facilities. You can experience all of these benefits and more by becoming a keto vegan practitioner today.

How to Get Started with the Keto Vegan Diet

There are two ways you can get started with a keto vegan diet. The first way is by simply jumping right in and cutting out all carbohydrates from your diet. This method can be quite shocking as the transition is very steep. However, the practitioner usually sees results in a quicker time frame and is less likely to deal with sugar withdrawal symptoms for a long period of time.

The second way involves slowly implementing keto vegan practices. This involves slowly reducing your carbohydrate consumption by progressively eating low amounts of carbs every day. The second way is less jarring to beginner practitioners and allows for a learning curve that is not so steep. While it can be easier for newbie keto vegan practitioners to follow the second method, it takes longer to see noticeable results.

The method that you choose to start the keto vegan diet is entirely up to you and depends on your goals and lifestyle. You can start by practicing one method, and then the other to see what works best for you.

No matter how you get started here are a few tips that are useful:

● Clear the non-keto vegan foods out of your cupboards and refrigerator and fill them up with keto-vegan friendly food so that you have an easier time sticking to this diet.

● Keep things simple at the beginning. Simply up your fat and protein intake and ensure that you are consuming less than 50 grams of carbohydrates every day without worrying too much about the comparative proportions of each. Adjust to the diet then worry about these later.

● Consult a licensed health care practitioner before you begin the keto vegan diet. Ensure that you do not have any preexisting medical conditions that might need addressing before you begin this diet.

Side Effects of the Keto Vegan Diet

Transitioning into a keto vegan lifestyle can be quite an adjustment and this has physical implications. It is not uncommon for new practitioners of the keto vegan diet to experience a condition known as the keto flu. Keto flu symptoms can include:

- Muscle cramps
- Low energy and weakness
- Dizziness
- Sleep disturbances
- Fatigue
- Poor concentration
- Diarrhea
- Constipation
- Nausea
- Headaches
- Irritability

The keto flu is typically experienced by people who jump right into this diet and follow all the rules off the bat. People who allow themselves to ease into this diet and lifestyle are less likely to experience the keto flu as the body is trained to slowly start burning more and more fat as carbohydrates are slowly removed from the diet.

The keto flu is typically caused by the alteration in water and mineral balances that the ketogenic vegan diet causes. You can restore this balance, and thereby curb the side effects of the keto flu, by adding more salt to your diet and taking mineral supplements such as sodium, potassium, and magnesium. These supplements are especially great at easing headaches, insomnia and muscle aches.

Additional supplements and substances that can aid in fighting the side effects of the keto flu include:

- Exogenous ketones. These are simply ketones that are synthesized outside your body. Taking the supplement increases blood ketone levels and therefore, helps fight keto flu.
- MCT oil. As mentioned earlier, this oil skips the digestive process and goes directly to the liver to be converted into ketones. This allows less of an adjustment period for your body to develop higher levels of ketones and thus, fights the symptoms of the keto flu. You can simply drink this oil as is or add it to your smoothies and other dishes
- Caffeine. Low energy is a common symptom of the keto flu and caffeine helps fight this symptom by boosting energy. Caffeine also increases athletic performance, increases fat loss, and reduces the risk of developing type 2 diabetes. You can increase the supply of caffeine in your diet by consuming unsweetened coffee and tea.

Other strategies that can be implemented to fight keto flu include staying hydrated, eating fiber-rich foods, engaging in light activity, and getting adequate rest.

Luckily, the symptoms of the keto flu typically only last for a few days and the practitioner can continue with his or her life without any negative consequence.

Exercising on the Keto Vegan Diet

Exercise and dieting go hand-in-hand if a person wants to live a healthy lifestyle and to lose weight in a safe and sustainable way. Experiencing the keto flu at the initial stages of starting this diet may make it difficult to partake in a normal exercise routine but long-term, practicing the keto vegan diet can actually improve your athletic performance, especially in endurance sports.

In the first few weeks of practicing the ketogenic vegan diet, it is recommended that you start with light exercises as your body begins to adjust to this fat-adapted way of eating. Such exercises include light hiking, walking, cycling, and yoga. It is also recommended that you stick to relatively flat surfaces as dizziness is a common symptom of the keto flu. No matter what exercise you choose to partake in or what stage in your ketogenic diet you are in be sure to be aware of your water intake so that you do not become dehydrated. You should also increase your mineral and electrolyte consumption accordingly to your level of exercise.

Chapter 2: What to Eat on Keto Vegan Diet

Foods That Should be Avoided on the Keto Vegan Diet

- Meat and poultry such as pork, beef, turkey, and chicken.
- Seafood like fish, shrimp, clams, scallops and mussels.
- Dairy products like milk, butter, and yogurt.
- Eggs including egg whites and egg yolks.
- Animal-based products like whey protein and honey.
- Fruits. Small amounts of some berries like raspberries and strawberries are allowed.
- Grains and starches like cereal, bread, baked goods, rice, pasta, and grains.
- Sugary drinks like sweet tea, soda, juice, fruit-based smoothies, sports drinks, and chocolate milk.
- Sugar-free drinks like diet soda. These are often high in sugar alcohols and are highly processed.
- Sweeteners like brown sugar, white sugar, agave, and maple syrup.
- Starchy root vegetables such as potatoes, sweet potatoes, winter squash, and beets.
- Beans and legumes like black beans, chickpeas, and kidney beans.
- Alcohol such as beer, sweetened cocktails, and wine. These do not need to be cut from the diet entirely, but they need to be severely limited.
- Common sauces and condiments like barbecue sauce, sweetened salad dressings, marinades, and ketchup. They often contain sugar and unhealthy fats.
- Highly processed foods. Packaged foods must be limited on the keto vegan diet.

Foods That You Can Eat on the Keto Vegan Diet

- Nuts and seeds such as chia seeds, pumpkin seeds, almonds, flax seeds, walnuts, sesame seeds, pistachios, Brazil nuts, and macadamia nuts.
- Nut and seed kinds of butter like peanut butter, almond butter, sunflower butter, cashew butter.
- Avocados. In addition to providing great fat content to this diet, avocados have large amounts of vitamins and minerals like potassium, which can help combat the keto flu.
- Coconut products like unsweetened coconut, coconut cream, full-fat coconut milk
- Healthy oils such as extra virgin olive oil, avocado oil and coconut oil.
- Vegetables with low carbohydrate content like onions, tomatoes, and peppers.
- Cruciferous vegetables such as broccoli, kale, zucchini, and cauliflower.
- Berries. Most fruits have a high sugar content and are thus excluded from this diet, but some berries are the exception. Berries blueberries, blackberries, raspberries and strawberries are low in carbohydrates and sugar.
- Condiments such as herbs, garlic, nutritional yeast, vinegar, pepper and salt.
- Dark chocolate. The dark chocolate must be constituted of at least 70% cocoa.
- Sweeteners like stevia, erythritol, and xylitol, which must be used in moderation.
- Vegan full-fat "dairy" like Coconut yogurt, vegan butter, cashew cheese and vegan cream cheese.
- Vegan protein sources such as tofu and tempeh.

Common Mistakes People Make on the Keto Vegan Diet and How to Avoid Them

Mistake #1 - Being unprepared to deal with keto flu

Many people do not realize that their bodies need some time to adjust to not just a diet but a lifestyle. Therefore, they are typically unprepared to deal with the symptoms of starting a keto vegan diet. Moving from metabolizing carbohydrates to metabolizing fats is a big shift for the body. While the symptoms of the keto flu are not life-threatening on their own, they can be uncomfortable to deal with. Therefore, do not allow the keto flu to catch you unawares. Keep your schedule light when you first begin this journey. Ensure that you are in a position to get adequate rest to compensate for low energy and tiredness. Keep plenty of fluid on hand and up your intake of electrolytes.

Mistake #2 - Increasing fat intake too quickly

Consuming more healthy fat is essential for ketosis to occur on the keto vegan diet. However, adding too much to your diet too soon can be detrimental to your health because it can cause digestive issues to arise. To avoid this, gradually increase your fat intake over time.

Mistake #3 – Consuming too much protein and not enough fat

The keto vegan diet is a moderate protein diet and thus consuming too much protein should be avoided because it interferes with the process of ketosis. Consuming too much protein can occur because we often reach for high protein sources like nuts when hunger strikes between meals. To ensure that you consume a moderate amount of protein throughout the day, carefully plan your meals and snacks to ensure that your diet remains high in fats, moderate in proteins and low in carbohydrates.

Mistake #4 – Consuming the wrong types of fat

There are different types of fat and some are healthier to consume than others. On the keto vegan diet, it is recommended that you consume monounsaturated and saturated fats because they are the type of fats that are readily used up in ketosis. These types of fats are found in oils like olive, canola, and avocado. On the other hand, polyunsaturated fats should only be consumed in limited quantities because they cause unhealthy weight gain, which can counteract the great benefits of practicing the keto vegan diet.

Mistake #5 – Not consuming enough salt

When the body uses ketones to obtain energy, the rate at which the kidneys secrete sodium (salt) increases. This decrease in salt levels can be detrimental to health. Therefore, to compensate for this, the practitioner of the keto vegan diet needs to up their salt intake. Doing this also helps combat the symptoms of keto flu.

Mistake #6 – Still eating overly processed foods

The quality of food you consume on the keto vegan diet matters just as much as consuming higher amounts of fat. Avoid processed foods even if they are low in carbohydrates because they can introduce other harmful substances to your body. This includes energy bars and diet sodas. Concentrate on consuming nutrient-rich, fresh foods as well as supplementing your diet with supplements like MCT oil.

Mistake #7 – Forgetting to indulge in other forms of self-care

The keto vegan diet helps in improving overall health, but you cannot limit your self-care to this diet. Self-care involves practicing routines that promote conditions that improve health. Practice other means of self-care like getting quality sleep, exercising, taking out quality 'me' time, and managing your stress levels. The combination of these self-care routines, in addition to practicing the keto vegan diet, helps develop overall well-being.

Mistake #8 – Becoming nutrient deficient

It is not uncommon for people who practice the keto vegan diet to have nutrient deficiencies because they do not ensure they have a balanced diet. Ensure that this does not happen to you by adding supplements like sodium, potassium, and magnesium to your diet.

Mistake #9 – Comparing yourself to other people

Everyone's body works differently. Some people see faster results on the keto vegan diet than others. You should not be discouraged if this happens to you. Also, you should not be overly focused on the numbers of the scale. This is a journey that you should enjoy. Therefore, you need to avoid comparing your progress to that of other people. Focus on the improvements you see and find encouragement to keep on going based on that progress.

Chapter 3: Meal Plan, Preparation and Storage

21-Day Keto Vegan Meal Plan

Day 1
Breakfast: Cashew Coconut Breakfast Bars
Lunch: Cucumber Tomato Salad
Dinner: Cauliflower Steaks
Snack 1: Lemon Squares
Snack 2: Raspberry Avocado Smoothie

Day 2
Breakfast: Cauliflower Berry Breakfast Bowl
Lunch: Oven Baked Spicy Cauliflower Wings
Dinner: Veggie Walnut Soup
Snack 1: Peanut Butter Energy Bars
Snack 2: Handful of Berries

Day 3
Breakfast: Breakfast Cereal with Almond Milk
Lunch: Spicy Cucumber Salad
Dinner: Roasted Red Pepper Soup
Snack 1: Raw Strawberry Crumble
Snack 2: Sliced cucumber topped with Cauliflower Hummus

Day 4
Breakfast: Breakfast Bagels with Pecan Butter
Lunch: Grilled Tofu Skewers
Dinner: Zucchini Spinach Ravioli
Snack 1: Cashew Yogurt topped with Chopped Almonds
Snack 2: Coconut Protein Crackers

Day 5
Breakfast: Cranberry Breakfast Bar
Lunch: Creamy Tomato Soup
Dinner: Keto Vegan Shepherd's Pie
Snack 1: Celery Sticks topped with Pecan Butter
Snack 2: Almond Cookies

Day 6
Breakfast: Pumpkin Spice Pancakes
Lunch: Avocado Zucchini Noodles
Dinner: Green Soup
Snack 1: Sliced Bell Peppers and Guacamole
Snack 2: Candied Toasted Cashew Nuts

Day 7
Breakfast: Lemon Pancakes
Lunch: Creamy Pumpkin Soup
Dinner: Portobello Mushroom Tacos with Guacamole

Snack 1: Coconut Fat Cups
Snack 2: Spiced Kale Chips

Day 8
Breakfast: Keto Vegan Vanilla French Toast
Lunch: Lime Coconut Cauliflower Rice
Dinner: Roasted Mushroom Burgers
Snack 1: Almond Coconut Fat Cups
Snack 2: Baked Zucchini Chips

Day 9
Breakfast: Cashew Yogurt Bowl
Lunch: Sautéed Jackfruit Cauliflower Bowl
Dinner: Roasted Radishes
Snack 1: Peanut Butter Cups
Snack 2: Handful of Raw Pumpkin Seeds

Day 10
Breakfast: Cinnamon Coconut Porridge
Lunch: Tuna Imitation Salad
Dinner: Roasted Pepper Zoodles
Snack 1: Coconut cream with Berries
Snack 2: Pitted Olives

Day 11
Breakfast: Zucchini Breakfast Bar
Lunch: Lettuce Salad Bowl
Dinner: Creamy Curry Zucchini Noodles
Snack 1: Keto Vegan Granola Mix
Snack 2: Toasted Coconut Chips

Day 12
Breakfast: Overnight Coconut Pumpkin Porridge
Lunch: Keto Vegan Empanada
Dinner: Creamy Spinach Shirataki
Snack 1: Macadamia Nut Bar
Snack 2: Celery Sticks and Almond Butter

Day 13
Breakfast: Cheesy Scrambled Tofu
Lunch: Avocado Fries
Dinner: Tempeh Broccoli Stir Fry Dinner
Snack 1: Cashew Coconut Bar
Snack 2: Handful of Raw Brazil Nuts

Day 14
Breakfast: Chocolate Waffles
Lunch: Sautéed Squash Kale Bowl
Dinner: Sautéed Brussel Sprouts Dish
Snack 1: Handful of Raw Macadamia Nuts
Snack 2: Coconut Milk Dairy-Free Yogurt

Day 15
Breakfast: Macadamia Nut Bar
Lunch: Avocado Cauliflower Salad
Dinner: Cauliflower Pizza Crust with Veggie Toppings
Snack 1: Flax Seed Crackers
Snack 2: Handful of Dried Coconut

Day 16
Breakfast: Spaghetti Squash Hashbrowns
Lunch: Avocado Cauliflower Salad
Dinner: Tofu Tomato Stir Fry
Snack 1: Apple Cider Donut
Snack 2: Blueberry Protein Smoothie

Day 17
Breakfast: Blueberry Scones
Lunch: Zucchini Veggie Wraps
Dinner: Walnut Zucchini Chili
Snack 1: Avocado Slices
Snack 2: Mint Cauliflower Smoothie

Day 18
Breakfast: Chocolate Zucchini Pancakes
Lunch: Cauliflower Cabbage Tortillas
Dinner: Roasted Veggies on Broccoli Rice
Snack 1: Seaweed Snacks
Snack 2: Handful of Cherry Tomatoes

Day 19
Breakfast: Avocado Breakfast Bowl
Lunch: Zucchini Green Bean Salad
Dinner: Falafel with Tahini Sauce
Snack 1: Vanilla Coconut Smoothie
Snack 2: Handful of Almonds

Day 20
Breakfast: 4 Seed Keto Vegan Bread with Strawberry Jam
Lunch: Cauliflower Pizza Bites
Dinner: Keto Vegan Thai Curry
Snack 1: Chocolate Avocado Smoothie
Snack 2: Handful of Peanuts

Day 21
Breakfast: Protein-Packed Blueberry Smoothie
Lunch: Tofu and Veggie Stir Fry
Dinner: Pesto Zucchini Noodles with Cherry Tomatoes
Snack 1: Avocado Fries
Snack 2: Handful of Cashew nuts

Keto Vegan Shopping List

One of the best things about preparing your own meals is having complete control of what goes into the dishes and therefore, what goes into your body. Good quality ingredients can make or break a dish. You need to get the best ingredients to not only keep your body within ketosis limits but to also make yourself feel good as well as look great. Luckily, I have made this easy for you. To help kick-start your keto vegan diet in the right way, I have compiled a shopping list that will take the hassle and headache out of figuring what to get at the grocery store.

Peruse the list below and simply eliminate items that are already in your kitchen cabinet and shop based on what you plan to prepare for that week or month. This will save you time, money, and energy.

Fruits (fresh, dried and frozen)

Avocados, berries (consumed in moderation), coconut, cranberries, lemon, lime, olives, tomatoes

Nuts and seeds

Almonds, Brazil nuts, cashew nuts (consumed in moderation), chia seeds, flax seeds, hazelnuts, hemp seeds, macadamia nuts, pecans, peanuts, pine nuts (consumed in moderation), pistachios (consumed in moderation), pumpkin seeds, sunflower seeds, walnuts

Nut and seed butters

Almond butter, coconut butter (also called the coconut manna), hazelnut butter, macadamia nut butter, peanut butter, pecan butter, sunflower seed butter, tahini, walnut butter

Vegetables

Artichoke hearts, arugula, asparagus, bell peppers, beets (consumed in moderation), bok choy, broccoli, Brussel sprouts (consumed in moderation), butternut squash, cabbage, carrots (consumed in moderation) cauliflower, celery, collards, cucumber, daikon radishes, eggplant, fennel, garlic, kale, lettuce, mushrooms, mustard greens, okra, onion (consumed in moderation), pumpkin, shallots, spinach, spaghetti squash, sprouts, turnips, zucchini

Dairy Alternatives

Cashew cheese, vegan butter, vegan cheeses, vegan cream cheese, vegan mayo

Sweeteners

Erythritol, liquid and powdered stevia, monk fruit sweetener

Spices

Bay leaf, black pepper, cayenne pepper, cinnamon, clove, coriander, cumin, curry powder, garlic powder, nutmeg, onion powder, paprika, salt, thyme, turmeric

Oils and Fats

Almond oil, avocado oil, cacao butter, coconut oil, flaxseed oil, hazelnut oil, macadamia nut oil, MCT oil, olive oil, walnut oil

Other Ingredients

Almond extract, almond flour, apple cider vinegar, baking powder, baking soda, balsamic vinegar, coconut aminos, coconut flour, coconut milk (canned and full fat), dairy-free yogurt such as cashew yogurt, dark chocolate (70% and up), jackfruit, kelp noodles, nutritional yeast, psyllium husk, seaweed snacks, seitan, shirataki noodles, soy sauce, tamari, tempeh, tofu, vanilla extract, white vinegar

Preparing and Storing Food on the Keto Vegan Diet

Food poisoning is a big concern no matter what diet you practice. Therefore, here are a few tips for ensuring that you not only prepare food that is safe and healthy to eat but you also store food in a way that extends this health and safety.

- Ensure that your hands are washed thoroughly before handling food. This prevents the transfer of bacteria and helps prevent sickness. Also, ensure that the work surface and equipment that you use to prepare and store food are cleaned before and after use.
- Keep food out of the food temperature danger zone. This zone is between 40 and 140 degrees Fahrenheit. Bacteria grows rapidly in this zone. Therefore, it is important to keep food out of this temperature zone.
- Take special care with high-risk foods. Food-poisoning bacteria thrive better on certain foods such as lasagna, curries, vegan dairy substitutes, prepared salads, sandwiches, mousse, and others. Therefore, special care needs to be taken to keep them out of the temperature danger zone.
- Ensure that your refrigerator and freezer is set to the correct temperature. In keeping with the food temperature zone, your refrigerator should be set to 40 degrees Fahrenheit or below. Your freezer should be 5 degrees Fahrenheit or lower.
- Transport frozen and chilled goods in the right way. After grocery shopping, place your chilled and frozen goods in an insulated cooler bag to keep them cold while moving them from the grocery store to your home. Keep them separated from warm and hot goods and place them in the refrigerator and freezer on immediate arrival at home.
- Store cooked food safely. Never place warm or hot food in the refrigerator or freezer as this increases the internal temperature of the appliance and potentially places not only that food item in the food temperature danger zone but all others in there as well. Allow food to cool completely first. Store food in the refrigerator or freezer by placing them in airtight containers or bags. It is also important that you store cooked food away from raw food to avoid the transfer of bacteria.
- When cooking food, ensure that all food is thoroughly cooked to kill any harmful bacteria.

Chapter 4: Sauces and Condiments Recipes

Sauces and condiments are great for adding flavor and variation to any dish. They are great for dipping fruits and vegetables, tossing salads, spreading on sandwiches and burgers, topping soups and more. Unfortunately, many traditional sauces and condiments contain high carb ingredients like sugar and/or animal-based products like eggs.

You are not confined to dishes that lack flavor on the ketogenic vegan diet, luckily. This section of the book provides recipes for sauces and condiments that will infuse your meals with flavor and variety, and they do so with ingredients that are both vegan and ketogenic friendly.

Keto Salsa Verde

Nutritional Information:
Total fat: 25.3g
Cholesterol: 0mg
Sodium: 475mg
Total carbohydrates: 0.8g
Dietary fiber: 0.3g
Protein: 0.2g
Calcium: 8mg
Potassium: 27mg
Iron:0mg
Vitamin D: 0mcg
Time: 5 minutes
Serving Size: 5
Ingredients:
- 4 tbsp fresh cilantro, finely chopped
- ¼ cup fresh parsley, finely chopped
- 2 garlic cloves, grated
- 2 tsp lemon juice
- ¾ cup of olive oil
- 2 tbsp small capers
- 1 tsp of salt
- ½ tsp black pepper

Directions:
1. Add all ingredients to a large mixing bowl. Can be mixed with by hand or with an immersion blender. Mix until desired consistency is achieved.
2. Can be served over burgers, sandwiches, salads and more. Can be stored in the refrigerator for up to 5 days or for longer in the freezer.

Chimichurri

Nutritional Information:

Total fat: 25.3g

Cholesterol: 0mg

Sodium: 3mg

Total carbohydrates: 1.6g

Dietary fiber: 0.3g

Protein: 0.3g

Calcium: 8mg

Potassium: 47mg

Iron: 0mg

Vitamin D: 0mcg

Time: 5 minutes

Serving Size: 8

Ingredients:
- ½ yellow bell pepper, deseeded and finely chopped
- 1 green chili pepper, deseeded and finely chopped
- Juice and zest of 1 lemon
- 1 cup olive oil
- ½ cup parsley, chopped
- 2 garlic cloves, grated
- Salt and pepper to taste

Directions:
1. Add all ingredients to a large mixing bowl. Can be mixed with by hand or with an immersion blender. Mix until desired consistency is achieved.
2. Can be served over burgers, sandwiches, salads and more. Can be stored in the refrigerator for up to 5 days or for longer in the freezer.

Keto Vegan Raw Cashew Cheese Sauce

Nutritional Information:

Total fat: 15.5g

Cholesterol: 0mg

Sodium: 34mg

Total carbohydrates: 9.23g

Dietary fiber: 1.6g

Protein: 5.1g

Calcium: 14mg

Potassium: 217mg

Iron: 2mg

Vitamin D: 0mcg

Time: 5 minutes

Serving Size: 6

Ingredients:
- 1 cup raw cashews, soaked in water for at least 3 hours prior to making recipe
- 2 tbsp olive oil
- 2 tbsp nutritional yeast
- ¼ tsp garlic powder
- 2 tbsp fresh lemon juice
- ½ cup water
- Salt to taste

Directions:
1. To prepare cashews prior to making the sauce, boil 2 cups of water turn off heat and add cashews. This can be allowed to soak overnight. Rinse and strained cashews. Discard water.
2. Add all ingredients to a food processor and blend until a smooth consistency is achieved. Can be used to make pizzas, over roasted veggies, in lasagna, as a dip and more.

Spicy Avocado Mayonnaise

Nutritional Information:
Total fat: 9.8g
Cholesterol: 0mg
Sodium: 23mg
Total carbohydrates: 4.6g
Dietary fiber: 3.4g
Protein: 1g
Calcium: 7mg
Potassium: 252mg
Iron: 0mg
Vitamin D: 0mcg
Time: 10 minutes
Serving Size: 8
Ingredients:
- 2 ripe avocados, pitted and peeled
- ¼ jalapeno pepper, minced
- 2 tbsp lemon juice
- ½ tsp onion powder
- 2 tbsp fresh cilantro, chopped
- Salt to taste

Directions:
1. Add all ingredients to a food processor and blender until a smooth creamy consistency is achieved. The jalapeno peppers can be foregone if you prefer a cooler mayo. Can be enjoyed in sandwiches, on toast, as a topping, in veggie wraps and in salads

Green Coconut Butter

Nutritional Information:
Total fat: 5.2g
Cholesterol: 0mg
Sodium: 3mg
Total carbohydrates: 1.7g
Dietary fiber: 1.2g
Protein: 0.7g
Calcium: 0mg
Potassium: 3mg
Iron: 0mg
Vitamin D: 0mcg
Time: 10 minutes
Serving Size: 18
Ingredients:
- 2 cups unsweetened shredded coconut
- 2 tsp matcha powder
- 1 tbsp coconut oil

Directions:
1. Add shredded coconut to a food processor and blend for 5 minutes or until a smooth but runny consistency is achieved.
2. Add matcha powder and olive oil. Blend for 1 more minute.
3. Can be stored in an airtight container at room temperature for up to 2 weeks. Makes a delicious fruit dip and can be added to smoothies, on pancakes and on toast.

Spiced Almond Butter

Nutritional Information:
Total fat: 9.5g
Cholesterol: 0mg
Sodium: 117mg
Total carbohydrates: 4.1g
Dietary fiber: 2.4g
Protein: 4g
Calcium: 52mg
Potassium: 140mg
Iron: 1mg
Vitamin D: 0mcg
Time: 10 minutes
Serving Size: 10
Ingredients:
- 2 cups raw almond
- ⅛ tsp allspice
- ⅛ tsp cinnamon
- ⅛ tsp cardamom
- ⅛ tsp ground ginger
- ⅛ tsp ground cloves
- ½ tsp salt

Directions:
1. Place all ingredients in a food processor and blend until a smooth consistency is achieved. Makes a delicious fruit and veggie dip and can be added to smoothies, on toast, on pancakes and waffles.

Keto Strawberry Jam

Nutritional Information:

Total fat: 0g
Cholesterol: 0mg
Sodium: 0mg
Total carbohydrates: 1g
Dietary fiber: 0.2g
Vitamin D: 0mcg
Time: 25 minutes

Protein: 0.1g
Calcium: 1mg
Potassium: 14mg
Iron: 0mg

Serving Size: 18

Ingredients:
- 1 cup fresh strawberries, chopped
- 1 tbsp lemon juice
- 4 tsp xylitol
- 1 tbsp water

Directions:
1. Add all ingredients to a small saucepan and place over medium heat. Stir to combine and cook for about 15 minutes. Stir occasionally.
2. After 15 minutes are up, mash-up strawberries with a potato masher or fork.
3. Pour into a heat-safe container such as a mason jar.
4. Allow to cool then cover with a lid and refrigerate. Can be stored in the refrigerator for up to 3 days. Goes great with toast and sweet sandwiches.

Chocolate Coconut Butter

Nutritional Information:

Total fat: 17.4g
Cholesterol: 0mg
Sodium: 17mg
Total carbohydrates: 0.9g
Dietary fiber: 0.6g
Time: 25 minutes
Serving Size: 20

Protein: 0.3g
Calcium: 0mg
Potassium: 0mg
Iron: 0mg
Vitamin D: 0mcg

Ingredients:
- ½ lb. unsweetened shredded coconut
- 3 tbsp cocoa butter
- ⅛ tsp salt

Directions:
Preheat your oven to 350 degrees F.
Place shredded coconut on a greased baking sheet. Spread out into a thin, even layer.
Bake for up to 15 minutes or until the coconut flakes are golden brown. Stir the coconut shreds every 3 minutes and watch them closely because they burn very easily and quickly.
Allow the coconut flakes to cool for 15 minutes.
Add coconut flakes to a food processor and blend until smooth and creamy yet runny in consistency.
Adding cocoa butter and salt and blend to incorporate well.
Pour into an airtight jar and seal lid. The consistency will thicken up as the butter cools. The oil may separate and float to the top of the container as the butter cools. Simply reheat a portion in the microwave just before using. Can be stored for up to a whole year at room temperature!

Orange Dill Butter

Nutritional Information:

Total fat: 1.5g

Cholesterol: 0mg

Sodium: 199mg

Total carbohydrates: 1g

Dietary fiber: 0.3g

Time: 15 minutes

Serving Size: 12

Protein: 0.1g

Calcium: 11mg

Potassium: 19mg

Iron: 0mg

Vitamin D: 0mcg

Ingredients:

- ½ cup vegan butter
- 2 tbsp fresh dill, finely chopped
- 2 tbsp orange zest
- 1 tsp salt

Directions:

1. Add 4 cups of water to a small pot and bring to a boil over high heat. Reduce heat to low and allow water to simmer.
2. Add vegan butter to a glass mason jar and screw on lid loosely.
3. Place mason jar in the boiling water. Ensure that the jar does not get submerged or over turn.
4. Allow the butter to melt and add remaining ingredients.
5. Remove the mason jar from the pot and allow to cool until the mixture becomes partially solidified.
6. Can be used alongside your favorite veggies to infuse them with flavor and fat. Can be stored in the refrigerator for up to 2 weeks.

Keto Caramel Sauce

Nutritional Information:

Total fat: 9.8g

Cholesterol: 0mg

Sodium: 29mg

Total carbohydrates: 4.6g

Dietary fiber: 0.7g

Time: 35 minutes

Serving Size: 8

Protein: 1.7g

Calcium: 6mg

Potassium: 90mg

Iron: 1mg

Vitamin D: 0mcg

Ingredients:

- ½ cup raw cashews
- ½ cup coconut cream, melted
- 10 drops liquid stevia
- 2 tbsp vegan butter
- 3 tsp vanilla extract
- A pinch of salt

Directions:

Preheat your oven to 325 degrees F

Place nuts on a greased baking tray and toast for 20 minutes or until lightly golden and crunchy. Allow the nuts to cool slightly then add to a food processor and blend to a slightly lumpy consistency.

Add remaining ingredients and blend until a smooth and creamy consistency is achieved. Do not over blend or the coconut cream will become separated from the rest of the ingredients.

Can be stored in a glass, airtight container in the refrigerator if not being served immediately. To reheat the caramel to make it more flowable, add to a saucepan and gently warm on low heat.

Can be served with your favorite keto vegan treats such as ice-cream.

Pecan Butter

Nutritional Information:
Total fat: 25g
Cholesterol: 0mg
Sodium: 0mg
Total carbohydrates: 5g
Dietary fiber: 3.8g
Protein: 3.8g
Calcium: 25mg
Potassium: 145mg
Iron: 1mg
Vitamin D: 0mcg
Time: 10 minutes
Serving Size: 8
Ingredients:
- 3 cups pecans, soaked well at least 3 hours, rinsed, strained and dried

Directions:
1. Add the pecans to a food processor and blend until a smooth and creamy consistency is achieved. Scrape down the sides of the bowl when necessary.
2. Transfer to a mason jar and store in the refrigerator. Can be stored in the refrigerator for several months. Makes a great spread on toast and sandwiches and a great fruit and veggie dip.

Keto Vegan Ranch Dressing

Nutritional Information:
Total fat: 11.9g
Cholesterol: 0mg
Sodium: 50mg
Total carbohydrates: 4.8g
Dietary fiber: 1.3g
Protein: 1.7g
Calcium: 79mg
Potassium: 223mg
Iron: 3mg
Vitamin D: 0mcg
Time: 5 minutes
Serving Size: 10
Ingredients:
- 1 cup vegan mayo
- 1 ½ cup coconut milk
- 2 scallions
- 2 garlic cloves, peeled
- 1 cup fresh dill
- 1 tsp garlic powder
- Salt and pepper to taste

Directions:
1. Add scallion, fresh dill and garlic cloves to a food processor and pulse until finely chopped.
2. Add the rest of the ingredients and blend until a smooth, creamy consistency is achieved. Makes a great creamy salad dressing. Store in the refrigerator.

Cauliflower Hummus

Nutritional Information:

Total fat: 2.7g

Cholesterol: 0mg

Sodium: 12mg

Total carbohydrates: 2.7g

Dietary fiber: 1.2g

Protein: 1.3g

Calcium: 11mg

Potassium: 138mg

Iron: 1mg

Vitamin D: 0mcg

Time: 20 minutes

Serving Size: 7

Ingredients:

- 1 large head cauliflower
- 1 tbsp almond butter
- 1 garlic clove, finely chopped
- 1 tbsp lemon juice
- 2 tsp olive oil
- ¼ tsp cumin
- Salt and pepper to taste

Directions:

1. Cut cauliflower into florets and place in a large microwave-safe bowl. Microwave for 10 minutes on high heat or until completely cooked through.
2. Transfer cauliflower florets to a food processor. Add the rest of the ingredients. Blend until smooth, creamy consistency is reached. Can be stored in the refrigerator in an airtight container for up to 5 days. Makes a great dip for fruits and veggies.

Cauliflower Cream

Nutritional Information:

Total fat: 0g

Cholesterol: 0mg

Sodium: 0mg

Total carbohydrates: 2.1g

Dietary fiber: 1g

Protein: 0.8g

Calcium: 9mg

Potassium: 121mg

Iron: 0mg

Vitamin D: 0mcg

Time: 10 minutes

Serving Size: 10

Ingredients:

- 4 cups cauliflower florets
- ½ cup of water
- ¼ tsp salt

Directions:

1. Add cauliflower, salt and water to a medium pan and place over high heat. Bring to a boil then reduce heat to low and allow to simmer for 12 minutes.
2. Allow the cauliflower mixture to cool for 10 minutes then transfer to a blender and blend until a smooth and creamy consistency is achieved. Can be used immediately or stored in the refrigerator in an airtight container for up to 2 days. Makes a great addition to soups casserole and even sweet treats like brownies.

Eggplant Dip

Nutritional Information:
Total fat: 6.1g
Cholesterol: 0mg
Sodium: 3mg
Total carbohydrates: 5.9g
Dietary fiber: 3.5g
Protein: 1.3g
Calcium: 27mg
Potassium: 222mg
Iron: 1mg
Vitamin D: 0mcg
Time: 40 minutes
Serving Size: 10
Ingredients:
- 2 large eggplants, cut lengthwise
- ½ tsp ground cumin
- ¼ cup olive oil
- 1 tbsp lemon juice
- 2 tbsp toasted sesame seeds
- Salt and pepper to taste

Directions:
1. Preheat your oven to 400 degrees F.
2. Prepare a baking sheet by lining it with parchment paper.
3. Sprinkle salt along the surface of the eggplants and place salt side up on baking sheet.
4. Bake for 30 minutes or until the eggplant is soft.
5. Allow eggplant to cool then peel the skin off and cut into cubes. Transfer to a blender.
6. Add cumin, olive oil, lemon juice and pepper and blend until a smooth and creamy consistency is achieved.
7. Transfer to a serving bowl and sprinkle with toasted sesame seeds. Makes a great dip for vegetables and a topping for sandwiches and burgers.

Chapter 5: Breakfast Recipes

Breakfast is often referred to as the most important meal of the day. This is with good reason because a nutrition-packed breakfast can give you that initial boost to optimize your physical and mental facilities so that you perform efficiently and productivity from the jump. Keto vegan breakfasts provide high fat and protein values while remaining low in carbs so that your body achieves and maintains ketosis. Therefore, not only are you performing at your best, but you gain all the benefits of veganism while managing your weight.

Cauliflower Berry Breakfast Bowl

Nutritional Information:
Total fat: 8g
Cholesterol: 0mg
Sodium: 40mg
Total carbohydrates: 13.8g
Dietary fiber: 7.1g
Protein: 4.3g
Calcium: 155mg
Potassium: 220mg
Iron: 3mg
Vitamin D: 0mcg
Time: 15 minutes
Serving Size: 6
Ingredients:
- ½ cup cauliflower, frozen
- ¼ cup zucchini, frozen
- 1 cup fresh spinach
- ½ cup frozen raspberries
- 1 cup unsweetened almond milk
- 2 tbsp almond butter
- 3 tbsp chia seeds
- 1 tsp ground cinnamon

Directions:
1. Add all ingredients to a blender. Place the frozen ingredients closest to the blades. Blend until smooth and creamy consistency is achieved and all the ingredients are well incorporated.
2. Divide the mixture between serving bowls. Can be topped with fresh raspberries and serve.

No - Fuss Breakfast Cereal

Nutritional Information:
Total fat: 18.7g
Cholesterol: 0mg
Sodium: 23mg
Total carbohydrates: 8g
Dietary fiber: 4.4g
Protein: 4.7g
Calcium: 62mg
Potassium: 124mg
Iron: 2mg
Vitamin D: 0mcg
Time: 35 minutes
Serving Size: 8
Ingredients:
- 1 cup unsweetened coconut flakes
- ½ cup raw pumpkin seeds
- ½ cup sunflower seeds
- ¼ cup chia seeds
- 1 tbsp toasted sesame seeds
- ¼ cup coconut oil
- 1 1/2 tsp vanilla extract
- A pinch of salt
- Coconut milk and fresh berries, like blackberries or blueberries for serving

Directions:
1. Preheat your oven to 300 degrees F.
2. Prepare a baking sheet by lining it with parchment paper.
3. In a large mixing bowl, add coconut flakes, pumpkin seeds, sunflower seeds, chia seeds, sesame seeds and salt. Mix well.
4. Add coconut oil and vanilla extract. Mix again.
5. Spread mixture onto prepared baking sheet in an even layer.
6. Bake for 20 minutes or until cereal golden brown. Stir halfway through.
7. Remove cereal from oven and allow cereal to cool to preference. Serve with coconut milk and berries.

Easy Breakfast Bagels

Nutritional Information:
Total fat: 13.7g
Cholesterol: 0mg
Sodium: 95mg
Total carbohydrates: 29.8g
Dietary fiber: 23.2g
Protein: 5.1g
Calcium: 125mg
Potassium: 247mg
Iron: 5mg
Vitamin D: 0mcg
Time: 1 hour
Serving Size: 12
Ingredients:
- 1 cup ground flax seed
- 1 cup tahini
- ½ cup psyllium husks
- 2 cup water
- 2 tsp baking powder
- A pinch of salt

Directions:
1. Preheat your oven to 375 degrees F.
2. Prepare a baking sheet by lining it with parchment paper.
3. Add flax seeds, psyllium husk, baking powder and salt to a bowl. Whisk to combine.
4. In a small bowl, whisk together water and tahini. Pour into dry ingredients and fold in. Knead to form the dough.
5. Create 12 circles about 4" in diameter, and 1/4" thick.
6. Place circles on prepared baking sheet, spaced equally apart. Cut a small circle from the middle of each circle.
7. Bake for around 40 minutes or until golden brown.
8. Remove from oven and allow to cool.
9. Cut in half and top as desired. Serve.

Cranberry Breakfast Bars

Nutritional Information:
Total fat: 15.7g
Cholesterol: 0mg
Sodium: 5mg
Total carbohydrates: 6.3g
Dietary fiber: 3.4g
Protein: 2.3g
Calcium: 49mg
Potassium: 151mg
Iron: 1mg
Vitamin D: 0mcg
Time: 55 minutes
Serving Size: 10
Ingredients:
- ⅓ cup dried cranberries
- 1 cup pecans
- 1 cup water
- ¼ cup coconut butter, softened
- 2 tbsp granulated erythritol
- 1 tbsp ground flax seed
- 2 tsp allspice blend
- 1 ½ tsp baking powder
- 1 tsp vanilla extract

Directions:
1. Preheat your oven to 350 degrees F.
2. Prepare an 8x8 brownie pan by lining it with parchment paper.
3. Add all ingredients to a blender and blend until slightly lumpy consistency is achieved.
4. Pour mixture into prepared brownie pan. Use a spatula to smooth the top.
5. Bake for 45 minutes or until a toothpick comes out clean when inserted into the center.
6. Remove the pan from the oven and allow to cool completely before removing and slicing into individual bars. If you do not allow the bars to cool completely then they will fall apart. Serve.

Pumpkin Spice Pancakes

Nutritional Information:
Total fat: 6.1g
Cholesterol: 0mg
Sodium: 3mg
Total carbohydrates: 5.9g
Dietary fiber: 3.5g
Protein: 1.3g
Calcium: 27mg
Potassium: 222mg
Iron: 1mg
Vitamin D: 0mcg
Time: 25 minutes
Serving Size: 6
Ingredients:
- ¼ cup pumpkin puree
- ⅓ cup almond milk
- ⅓ cup coconut flour
- ⅓ cup water
- ⅓ cup almond flour
- ¼ tsp baking soda
- 1 tbsp vanilla protein powder
- ⅛ tsp ground cinnamon
- ⅛ tsp ground ginger
- 1 tsp stevia powder

Directions:
1. Add coconut flour, almond flours, baking soda, cinnamon, ginger, stevia and protein powder to a mixing bowl. Mix well.
2. Add almond milk, water and pumpkin puree to a blender and blend to a smooth consistency. Pour into dry ingredients and combine until no lumps are visible.
3. Grease a nonstick skillet and place on medium heat. Add 1/4 cup of batter to heated skillet at a time. Cook for 1 minute or until the bottom edges turn golden brown. Flip and cook for 1 more minute. Repeat until all batter is used up.
4. Remove, plate and serve with toppings such as fresh berries or berry jam.

Lemon Pancakes

Nutritional Information:
Total fat: 18.5g
Cholesterol: 0mg
Sodium: 52mg
Total carbohydrates: 16.6g
Dietary fiber: 11.2g
Protein: 2.7g
Calcium: 29mg
Potassium: 80mg
Iron: 1mg
Vitamin D: 0mcg
Time: 1 hour
Serving Size: 6
Ingredients:
- ½ tsp vanilla extract
- 1 tbsp lemon juice
- 2 tbsp coconut butter, melted
- 1 tbsp granulated erythritol
- 5 tbsp almond milk
- ¼ cup coconut flour
- ½ tsp baking powder
- 1 tbsp psyllium husk
- A pinch of salt

Directions:
1. In a medium mixing bowl, whisk together coconut flour, baking powder, salt and psyllium.
2. In a large mixing bowl, whisk together remaining ingredients then stir into dry mixture. Combine thoroughly and ensure that there are no lumps.
3. Allow the mixture to sit for 5 minutes or until a stiff dough forms. You should be able to mold this dough with your hands. If not, stir in additional coconut flour.
4. Divide the dough into 5 equal portions to form 5 balls.
5. Heat a nonstick skillet over medium heat. Grease with coconut oil.
6. Flatten dough and add to pan. Cook for 5 minutes on each side or until golden brown and cooked through.
7. Allow to cool for a few minutes and serve.

Keto Vegan Vanilla French Toast

Nutritional Information:
Total fat: 8.3g
Cholesterol: 0mg
Sodium: 11mg
Total carbohydrates: 23.5g
Dietary fiber: 2.6g
Protein: 3.9g
Calcium: 12mg
Potassium: 166mg
Iron: 1mg
Vitamin D: 0mcg
Time: 20 minutes
Serving Size: 5
Ingredients:
- 5 slices fresh coconut bread (or any other keto vegan friendly sandwich bread)
- ¼ tsp ground cinnamon
- ¼ cup vanilla protein powder
- ½ cup almond milk
- A pinch of ground nutmeg

Directions:
1. Whisk together almond milk, protein powder, nutmeg and cinnamon in a shallow but wide dish that the bread can fit into. Ensure that there are no lumps in the mix.
2. Heat a nonstick skillet over medium heat and grease with coconut oil.
3. Soak each piece of bread in the vanilla protein powder mixture for 5 seconds on each side.
4. Place the soaked pieces of bread in the skillet and cook for 5 minutes so that the bottom turns golden brown. Flip and cook for another 5 minutes or until the other side is golden brown.
5. Plate and serve.

Cashew Yogurt Bowl

Nutritional Information:
Total fat: 11.4g
Cholesterol: 0mg
Sodium: 18mg
Total carbohydrates: 15.6g
Dietary fiber: 7.5g
Protein: 6.6g
Calcium: 180mg
Potassium: 170mg
Iron: 3mg
Vitamin D: 0mcg
Time: 5 minutes
Serving Size: 2
Ingredients:
- ¾ cup vegan cashew yogurt
- 1 tbsp flaxseed
- 1 tbsp chia seeds
- 1 tbsp hemp seed
- ¼ cup frozen blueberries

Directions:
1. Add the cashew yogurt to the bottom of the serving bowl.
2. Top with the remaining ingredients, going around steadily in a circle until all the ingredients are used up. Serve.

Cinnamon Coconut Porridge

Nutritional Information:

Total fat: 31.5g

Cholesterol: 0mg

Sodium: 8mg

Total carbohydrates: 9.8g

Dietary fiber: 9g

Protein: 21.7g

Calcium: 49mg

Potassium: 95mg

Iron: 11mg

Vitamin D: 0mcg

Time: 5 minutes

Serving Size: 1

Ingredients:

- 2 tbsp shredded coconut
- 1 tbsp ground flax seeds
- 2 tbsp hemp hearts
- ⅛ tsp cinnamon
- ⅛ tsp stevia powder
- ½ cup of boiling water
- Fresh mixed berries to top

Directions:

1. Add all ingredients except for fresh mixed berries and water to a serving bowl and stir to combine.
2. Add boiling water. Stir.
3. Allow the porridge to sit until it reaches a suitable eating temperature. The porridge will thicken as it cools down. Top with fresh mixed berries and serve.

Zucchini Breakfast Bars

Nutritional Information:

Total fat: 17g

Cholesterol: 0mg

Sodium: 35mg

Total carbohydrates: 10g

Dietary fiber: 6.3g

Protein: 7.1g

Calcium: 56mg

Potassium: 77mg

Iron: 3mg

Vitamin D: 0mcg

Time: 45 minutes

Serving Size: 6

Ingredients:

- 1 cup zucchini grated
- ¼ cup coconut butter, softened
- 2 tsp cinnamon
- 1 tbsp chia seeds
- ½ cup hemp hearts
- 2 tbsp granulated erythritol
- A pinch of salt

Directions:

1. Preheat your oven to 375 degrees F.
2. Prepare a 9 x 13 loaf pan by lining it with parchment paper.
3. To a large mixing bowl, add coconut butter, zucchini and erythritol. Combine thoroughly
4. Add the rest of the ingredients and stir to thoroughly incorporate. Allow the mixture to sit for 5 minutes so that the chia seeds thicken the batter.
5. Pour mixture into prepared pan and smooth top with a spatula.
6. Bake for 35 minutes or until the bars are golden brown and firm to the touch.
7. Allow to cool for at least 30 minutes before removing from the. Slice into individual bars and serve.

Overnight Coconut Pumpkin Porridge

Nutritional Information:

Total fat: 46g

Cholesterol: 0mg

Sodium: 313mg

Total carbohydrates: 16.9g

Dietary fiber: 9.8g

Protein: 11.4g

Calcium: 134mg

Potassium: 515mg

Iron: 6mg

Vitamin D: 0mcg

Time: 10 minutes

Serving Size: 2

Ingredients:

- 2 tsp of shredded coconut
- ½ cup coconut cream at room temperature
- 8 drops liquid stevia
- 2 tsp powdered stevia
- ½ cup almond milk
- 1 tsp hemp hearts
- 2 tbsp raw pumpkin seeds
- 1 tsp chia seeds
- ¼ tsp salt
- 1 tsp ground cinnamon
- 8 walnuts, halved

Directions:

1. In a small bowl, combine pumpkin seeds, chia seeds, hemp hearts, salt and half of cinnamon.
2. In another small bowl, whisk together almond milk and coconut cream. Pour this mixture into the seed mixture and stir to combine. Cover the resulting mixture and chill overnight.
3. When it is time to serve, heat the porridge in the microwave for 1 minute or in a saucepan over medium heat for 4 minutes or until warmed through.
4. Add remaining cinnamon, liquid stevia and powdered cinnamon stevia to mixture and mix. If the porridge is too thick, add more almond milk until desired consistency is reached.
5. Top with walnuts and shredded coconut and serve.

Cheesy Scrambled Tofu

Nutritional Information:
Total fat: 18.8g
Cholesterol: 0mg
Sodium: 418mg
Total carbohydrates: 9.6g
Dietary fiber: 3.3g
Protein: 10.9g
Calcium: 215mg
Potassium: 373mg
Iron: 3mg
Vitamin D: 0mcg
Time: 15 minutes
Serving Size: 4
Ingredients:

- 14 oz firm tofu
- 1 ½ tbsp nutritional yeast
- 3 oz vegan cheddar cheese
- 1 medium tomato, diced
- 1 cup spinach
- ½ tsp salt
- ½ tsp turmeric
- ½ tsp garlic powder
- 3 tbsp olive oil
- 2 tbsp yellow onion, diced

Directions:

1. Wrap the block of tofu in a clean cloth towel and gently squeeze to remove excess moisture. Set aside.
2. Place a nonstick skillet over medium heat. Add 1/3 of the olive oil and add onions. Sauté until the onions become translucent.
3. Add the block of tofu to the skillet and crumble using a fork or potato masher. Do this until the tofu resembles scrambled eggs.
4. Add the remaining oil, nutritional yeast, garlic powder, turmeric and salt and stir.
5. Cover the pot and continue to cook, stirring occasionally, until most of the moisture in the pot has evaporated.
6. Add spinach, tomato and vegan cheese. Cook for 1 more minute or until the spinach has wilted and the cheese is melted. Serve hot. Can be stored in the refrigerator for up to three days in an airtight container.

Chocolate Waffles

Nutritional Information:
Total fat: 58.3g
Cholesterol: 0mg
Sodium: 93mg
Total carbohydrates: 22.4g
Dietary fiber: 15.9g
Protein: 1.3g
Calcium: 32mg
Potassium: 168mg
Iron: 1mg
Vitamin D: 0mcg
Time: 25 minutes
Serving Size: 4
Ingredients:
- 3 tbsp cocoa powder
- ½ cup coconut flour
- ¼ cup coconut oil, softened
- 1 cup coconut milk at room temperature
- ½ teaspoon baking powder
- 3 tbsp granulated erythritol
- 2 tbsp psyllium husk
- A pinch of salt

Directions:
1. Preheat your waffle iron according to manufacturer's instructions.
2. Add cocoa powder, coconut flour, granulated erythritol, baking powder, salt and psyllium to a medium bowl. Stir to combine.
3. Add coconut oil to the dry mixture and stir until a stiff dough forms.
4. Add coconut milk in increments. Stir to fully incorporate before next addition. Once the milk has been added completely, let the mixture sit for 3 minutes so that it sets.
5. Divide the dough into 4 equal portions and make waffles according to waffle iron instructions. Allow to cool for a few minutes before serving.

Macadamia Nut Bars

Nutritional Information:
Total fat: 19.7g
Cholesterol: 0mg
Sodium: 4mg
Total carbohydrates: 3.6g
Dietary fiber: 2.3g
Protein: 1.6g
Calcium: 7mg
Potassium: 38mg
Iron: 1mg
Vitamin D: 0mcg
Time: 5 minutes
Serving Size: 8
Ingredients:
● 1/2 cup macadamia nuts
● 6 tbsp unsweetened shredded coconut
● 10 drops liquid stevia
● ¼ cup coconut oil
● ½ cup almond butter
Directions:
1. Prepare a 9x9 baking sheet by lining it with parchment paper.
2. Add macadamia nuts to a food processor and process until a fine meal consistency is achieved.
3. Combine shredded coconut, coconut oil and almond butter in a large mixing bowl.
4. Add macadamia nuts and the stevia drops.
5. Mix batter thoroughly.
6. Paul into the prepared baking sheet and refrigerate overnight. Slice into individual bars and serve.

Spaghetti Squash Hashbrowns

Nutritional Information:
Total fat: 7.2g
Cholesterol: 0mg
Sodium: 7mg
Total carbohydrates: 5.2g
Dietary fiber: 2.4g
Protein:0.9g
Calcium: 12mg
Potassium: 208mg
Iron: 0mg
Vitamin D: 0mcg
Time: 35 minutes
Serving Size: 10
Ingredients:
- 1 spaghetti squash
- 3 tbsp avocado oil
- ⅛ teaspoon sage, diced
- Salt and pepper to taste

Directions:
1. Wash and dry the spaghetti squash then cut into two halves. Using a knife, pierce the spaghetti squash several times.
2. Place in a shallow microwave-safe dish and add 1 inch of water. Microwave in 2 minute intervals for up to 8 minutes or until the squash becomes soft enough to pierce easily with a knife.
3. Allow the squash to become cool enough to handle then scoop out the seeds and stringy pieces. Shred with fork and place spaghetti strands in a bowl.
4. Add salt, pepper and sage to spaghetti squash. Mix well.
5. Form into 10 compact balls with your hand then press down into 1/2 inch thick hash brown patties. Use a paper towel to squeeze out any excess moisture from patties.
6. Place a nonstick skillet over medium heat and add avocado oil. When the oil is hot, add as many patties as the pan can carry to fry. Cook for 5 minutes or until underside is golden brown and the Patty is heated all the way through. Flip and cook for another 5 minutes or until the next side is golden brown as well.
7. Repeat with any remaining patties.
8. Allow to cool for a few minutes and serve with your favorite keto vegan friendly sauce or dip.

Blueberry Scones

Nutritional Information:
Total fat: 3g
Cholesterol: 0mg
Sodium: 30mg
Total carbohydrates: 2.4g
Dietary fiber: 0.9g
Protein: 1.2g
Calcium: 19mg
Potassium: 58mg
Iron: 0mg
Vitamin D: 0mcg
Time: 40 minutes
Serving Size: 6
Ingredients:
- ¼ cup fresh blueberries
- 1 cup almond flour
- ½ tsp baking powder
- ⅛ tsp powdered stevia
- ½ tbsp ground flax seed
- 1 ½ tbsp water
- 1 tbsp almond milk
- A pinch of salt

Directions:
1. Preheat your oven to 375 degrees F.
2. Prepare a baking sheet by lining it with parchment paper.
3. Create an egg substitute by mixing flaxseed and water in a small bowl. Set aside for 5 minutes.
4. In a large bowl, sift together almond flour, stevia, baking powder and salt.
5. Add blueberries to dry mixture. Mix to coat with dry mixture.
6. Combine egg substitute and almond milk in a small bowl. Pour into dry mixture and stir until fully incorporated. A soft dough should be created.
7. Shape 6 scones with 1/2 inch thickness and place on prepared baking sheet.
8. Bake for 20 minutes or until golden brown.
9. Remove and allow to cool for at least 10 minutes before serving.

Chocolate Zucchini Pancakes

Nutritional Information:
Total fat: 13.3g
Cholesterol: 0mg
Sodium: 11mg
Total carbohydrates: 11.3g
Dietary fiber: 5.2g
Protein: 5.2g
Calcium: 39mg
Potassium: 167mg
Iron: 2mg
Vitamin D: 0mcg
Time: 20 minutes
Serving Size: 4
Ingredients:
- 2 tbsp dark chocolate chips
- ¼ cup zucchini, shredded
- ½ cup almond flour
- 2 tbsp coconut flour
- 2 tbsp granulated erythritol
- ½ tsp baking powder
- 3 tbsp flaxseed
- ½ cup water
- 1 tsp of cinnamon
- ¼ cup almond milk

Directions:
1. Make egg substitute by combining flaxseed and water. Set aside for 5 minutes.
2. Add flax egg along with all of the ingredients except for chocolate chips to a blender. Blend until just combined or to a thick, pourable mixture.
3. Allow batter to sit for 10 minutes. Just before cooking, stir in chocolate chips.
4. Place a nonstick skillet oiled with a small bit of avocado or olive oil over medium heat. Pour small portions of batter into the heated pan. Cook for 3 minutes or until edges are golden brown. Flip and cook for another 3 minutes.
5. Repeat with any remaining. Serve warm.

Avocado Breakfast Bowl

Nutritional Information:
Total fat: 17.4g
Cholesterol: 2mg
Sodium: 28mg
Total carbohydrates: 11.4g
Dietary fiber: 5.6g
Protein: 6.5g
Calcium: 110mg
Potassium: 550mg
Iron: 2mg
Vitamin D: 0mcg
Time: 5 minutes
Serving Size: 3
Ingredients:
- 1 avocado, peeled and deseeded
- ¼ cup fresh spinach
- ¼ cup fresh mint
- 1 cup full fat coconut milk
- ¼ cup water
- 1 medium cucumber, peeled and chopped
- ½ scoop vanilla protein powder
- 2 tbsp apple cider vinegar
- 2 tbsp fresh lemon juice
- ½ cup ice cubes

Directions:
1. Add all ingredients except for the mixed berries to a blender and blend until a thick, smooth and creamy consistency is achieved.
2. Divide the mixture between serving bowls and top with fresh mixed berries or other toppings such as toasted coconut flakes, sesame seeds or pumpkin seeds. Serve immediately.

4 Seed Keto Vegan Bread

Nutritional Information:

Total fat: 10.9g

Cholesterol: 0mg

Sodium: 132mg

Total carbohydrates: 5.4g

Dietary fiber: 3.3g

Time: 1 hour 20 minutes

Protein: 4.5g

Calcium: 28mg

Potassium: 148mg

Iron: 3mg

Vitamin D: 0mcg

Serving Size: 18

Ingredients:

- ½ cup chia seeds
- ½ cup flax seeds
- 1 cup raw sunflower seeds
- 1 ½ cup raw pumpkin seeds
- ½ cup whole psyllium husk
- 1 tsp salt
- A pinch of powdered stevia
- 3 tbsp sunflower oil
- 1 ½ cup of warm water

Directions:

Preheat your oven to 350 degrees F.

Prepare a 1-pound loaf pan and a baking sheet by lining them with parchment paper.

Add pumpkin seeds to a food processor and process until finely chopped to a medium coarse flour consistency.

Transfer pumpkin seed flour to a medium mixing bowl. Add chia seeds, flax seeds, sunflower seeds, stevia and psyllium husks. Stir to mix.Stir in warm water and olive oil to form a uniform batter.Transfer batter into prepared loaf pan. Press into a uniform loaf with your hands. Bake for 45 minutes.

Remove the loaf pan from the oven and remove loaf. Place the loaf onto the prepared baking sheet so that the top is down and return it to the oven to bake for 15 more minutes or until tapping the top produces a hollow sound.

Remove from the oven and cool completely before slicing. Serve. Can be topped with your favorite keto vegan jam, avocado slices, nut butter and more when served. Can be stored in the refrigerator in an airtight container up to 7 days. Can be stored in the freezer for longer.

Cashew Coconut Breakfast Bars

Nutritional Information:

Total fat: 8.8g

Cholesterol: 0mg

Sodium: 3mg

Total carbohydrates: 5.7g

Dietary fiber: 3.5g

Time: 10 minutes

Protein: 1.8g

Calcium: 30mg

Potassium: 104mg

Iron: 1mg

Vitamin D: 0mcg

Serving Size: 25

Ingredients:

- 2 cups raw cashews
- 2 tbsp unsweetened shredded coconut
- 1 cup raw almonds
- 1 cup almond butter
- ¼ cup chia seeds
- Full fat coconut milk

Directions:

Prepare an 8x8 freezer-safe dish with parchment paper.

Add cashews and almonds to a food processors and process to form a crumbly texture.

Add almond butter and chia seeds and blend to form a sticky batter. If the batter is too thick, add coconut milk gradually until desired texture is achieved.

Pour cashew mixture into prepared freezer-safe dish and smooth into an even layer. Sprinkle with coconut flakes and place in freezer for at least 2 hours. Slice and serve. Keep frozen to store.

Chapter 6: Lunch Recipes

It is a common occurrence for people to skip lunch. This can be for a variety of reasons such as rushing to class, being buried in paperwork, trying to meet a deadline or having tons of errands to do that day. We often believe that we can gain time throughout the day by skipping this vital meal but that is not the case. Taking a lunch break actually helps you accomplish more because it allows your brain to switch off and regroup so that it can perform better.

Skipping lunch is a bad habit because it has detrimental effects on your overall health. Eating lunch is what gives you energy to keep plowing on through the day so that you cut through your to-do list. It helps you stay focused to perform at your best.

In addition, skipping lunch tends to lead to overeating at dinner time to compensate for the missed meal. This can lead to unhealthy weight gain.

Also, eating lunch helps improve the workings of your digestive system as it helps prevent bloating, acid reflux and indigestion.

Not only is eating lunch important for your physical, mental and emotional health, but it also helps you socialize more as it forces you to take a step back from your commitments and sit with other people so that you can have small talk or deeper conversations. Socialization is very important to healthy human development.

Below you can find a list of time-saving, good-for-your gut, tasty recipes that you can prepare in advance so that you have a healthy lunchtime meal rather than reaching for unhealthy convenience dishes. Preparing your own lunch helps you save time and money.

Quick and Easy Cucumber Tomato Salad

Nutritional Information:
Total fat: 16.5g
Cholesterol: 0mg
Sodium: 9mg
Total carbohydrates: 13.3g
Dietary fiber: 6.8g
Protein: 2.9g
Calcium: 30mg
Potassium: 662mg
Iron: 1mg
Vitamin D: 0mcg
Time: 15 minutes
Serving Size: 4
Ingredients:
- 1 large cucumber, skinned and chopped
- 1 ½ cup cherry tomatoes, quartered
- 2 ripe avocados, pitted, peeled and chopped into large chunks
- 1 green bell pepper, chopped
- 2 tbsp fresh cilantro chopped
- ½ tbsp avocado oil
- 1 tbsp red wine vinegar
- 1 tbsp almond
- Salt and pepper to taste

Directions:
1. Add all veggies to a large mixing bowl.
2. Whisk together almond oil, red wine vinegar, lemon juice, cilantro, salt and pepper to make vinaigrette.
3. Pour into veggies and toss to coat. Divide the salad among serving bowls and serve.

Oven Baked Spicy Cauliflower Wings

Nutritional Information:
Total fat: 1.1g
Cholesterol: 0mg
Sodium: 284mg
Total carbohydrates: 4.9g
Dietary fiber: 2.3g
Protein: 2g
Calcium: 19mg
Potassium: 264mg
Iron: 0mg
Vitamin D: 0mcg
Time: 45 minutes
Serving Size: 5
Ingredients:
- 4 cups cauliflower florets
- 3 tbsp hot sauce
- 1 tbsp almond flour
- 1 tbsp avocado oil
- Salt to taste

Directions:
1. Preheat your oven to 350 degrees F.
2. Prepare a baking sheet by lining it with parchment paper.
3. Mix all the ingredients in a medium mixing bowl and toss to thoroughly cut the cauliflower florets.
4. Place the cauliflower in a single layer on the prepared baking sheet.
5. Bake for 40 minutes or until the cauliflower is crisp at the edges. Turn the cauliflower halfway through the baking process. Serve warm with extra hot sauce if desired. Hot sauce can be removed from the recipe if you would like a milder flavor.

Spicy Cucumber Salad

Nutritional Information:
Total fat: 9.5g
Cholesterol: 0mg
Sodium: 404mg
Total carbohydrates: 5.7g
Dietary fiber: 1g
Protein: 1.6g
Calcium: 31mg
Potassium: 205mg
Iron: 1mg
Vitamin D: 0mcg
Time: 40 minutes
Serving Size: 3
Ingredients:
- 1 large cucumber, sliced
- 2 scallions, finely sliced
- 2 tbsp sesame oil
- ½ tsp toasted sesame seeds
- 1 tbsp rice vinegar
- 2 tbsp of low sodium soy sauce
- ½ tsp red pepper flakes, crushed
- Salt and pepper to taste

Directions:
1. In a small bowl, combine sesame oil, sesame seeds, rice vinegar, soy sauce, red pepper flakes, salt and pepper to create salad dressing.
2. Add cucumber and scallions to a mixing bowl and toss with salad dressing.
3. Refrigerate for at least 30 minutes to let the flavors marinade. Serve chilled.

Grilled Tofu Skewers

Nutritional Information:
Total fat: 3.8g
Cholesterol: 0mg
Sodium: 211mg
Total carbohydrates: 9.4g
Dietary fiber: 2.4g
Protein: 3.3g
Calcium: 61mg
Potassium: 385mg
Iron: 1mg
Vitamin D: 0mcg
Time: 35 minutes
Serving Size: 6

Ingredients:
- 1 block firm tofu
- 1 red bell pepper, cut into squares
- 1 yellow bell pepper, cut into squares
- 1 red onion, cut into squares
- 2 small zucchini, sliced
- 2 cups cherry tomatoes
- 2 tbsp low sodium soy sauce
- 2 tsp sesame seeds
- 3 tsp olive oil
- Salt and pepper to taste

Directions:
1. Press the tofu to extract any liquid for about half an hour and cut into cubes. Marinade in the soy sauce for 15 minutes.
2. While the tofu marinades, prepare veggies. Ensure that they are cut into the same size to ensure even cooking.
3. Assemble skewers by sticking vegetables and tofu cubes on bamboo sticks alternately until all the vegetables have been used.
4. Heat a grill or pan until sizzling hot. Grease with olive oil and place skewers on. Cook for a few minutes on each side until the vegetables are soft but not mushy, the peppers begin to char, and the tofu becomes golden brown. Season with salt and pepper, brush with olive oil and sprinkle with sesame seeds at the end of the cooking process.
5. Remove from grill or pan and serve hot with your favorite vegan keto friendly condiment.

Creamy Tomato Soup

Nutritional Information:
Total fat: 0.3g
Cholesterol: 0mg
Sodium: 10mg
Total carbohydrates: 5.6g
Dietary fiber: 1.8g
Protein: 1.3g
Calcium: 22mg
Potassium: 323mg
Iron: 1mg
Vitamin D: 0mcg
Time: 35 minutes
Serving Size: 10
Ingredients:
- 3 15-oz cans diced tomatoes with juice
- 3 ½ cup water
- 3 scallions, chopped
- 1 garlic clove, minced
- 1 tsp dried oregano
- 6 basil leaves
- ½ tsp smoked paprika
- Salt and pepper to taste

Directions:
1. Add all ingredients to a large pot and stir. Place over high heat and bring to a boil.
2. Reduce heat to medium low and simmer for 20 minutes or until the sauce thickens.
3. Can be served as is or an immersion blender can be used to achieve a smoother consistency. Separate into serving bowls and serve.

Avocado Zucchini Noodles

Nutritional Information:

Total fat: 31.7g

Cholesterol: 0mg

Sodium: 26mg

Total carbohydrates: 16.8g

Dietary fiber: 9.2g

Protein: 6.5g

Calcium: 53mg

Potassium: 997mg

Iron: 2mg

Vitamin D: 0mcg

Time: 15 minutes

Serving Size: 2

Ingredients:

- 1 medium zucchini
- 1 small avocado
- 1 cup cherry tomatoes, sliced
- ⅓ cup water
- 1 cup basil
- 2 tbsp lemon juice
- 4 tbsp pine nuts

Directions:

1. To make the zucchini noodles, use a spiralizer or peeler.
2. Add all the other ingredients except the cherry tomato to a blender and blend until a smooth creamy consistency is attained.
3. Transfer mixture to a large mixing bowl. Add zucchini noodles and tomatoes. Mix to combine. Serve. Can be stored in an airtight container in the refrigerator for up to 2 days.

Creamy Pumpkin Soup

Nutritional Information:

Total fat: 15.5g

Cholesterol: 0mg

Sodium: 1281mg

Total carbohydrates: 12.2g

Dietary fiber: 6.2g

Protein: 2.4g

Calcium: 27mg

Potassium: 244mg

Iron: 2mg

Vitamin D: 0mcg

Time: 20 minutes

Serving Size: 5

Ingredients:

- 1 15-oz can pumpkin puree
- ½ cup unsweetened coconut milk
- 2 tsp unsweetened Thai red curry paste
- ½ tsp salt
- ½ tsp onion powder
- ½ tsp garlic powder
- Water, if needed

Directions:

1. Add all ingredients to a medium pot and place over high heat. Bring to a boil while stirring constantly. Add water if needed to reach the desired consistency.
2. Reduce heat to low, cover the pot and allow to simmer for 10 minutes, stirring at 3 minutes intervals. Serve.

Lime Coconut Cauliflower Rice

Nutritional Information:
Total fat: 12.1g
Cholesterol: 0mg
Sodium: 97mg
Total carbohydrates: 8.6g
Dietary fiber: 4.3g
Protein: 8.8g
Calcium: 13mg
Potassium: 164mg
Iron: 2mg
Vitamin D: 0mcg
Time: 15 minutes
Serving Size: 2
Ingredients:
- 1 cup cauliflower florets
- 1 tbsp lime juice
- ½ cup full fat coconut milk
- ¼ cup hulled hemp seeds
- A pinch of salt

Directions:
1. To make a cauliflower rice, add cauliflower to food processor and pulse until a rice-like consistency is achieved.
2. Add riced cauliflower to a Dutch oven placed over medium heat. Stir in remaining ingredients except for lime juice.
3. Cover and cook for 10 minutes or until the liquid has evaporated from hemp seeds and the cauliflower rice is tender.
4. Remove from heat and allow to cool slightly and stir in lime juice. Serve.

Sautéed Jackfruit Cauliflower Bowl

Nutritional Information:
Total fat: 15.4g
Cholesterol: 0mg
Sodium: 172mg
Total carbohydrates: 13.6g
Dietary fiber: 6.6g
Protein: 5.3g
Calcium: 37mg
Potassium: 375mg
Iron: 1mg
Vitamin D: 0mcg
Time: 20 minutes
Serving Size: 4
Ingredients:
- 1 can jackfruit in water, drained and chopped
- 3 cups cauliflower rice
- 1 cup kale
- 1 tbsp chili powder
- 1 tbsp olive oil
- 1 tsp garlic powder
- 1 tsp onion powder
- Avocado slices for serving

Directions:
1. Add olive oil to a nonstick skillet and place over medium heat. Once it is heated and all the other ingredients except for the avocado.
2. Sauté until the cauliflower rice is tender. Stir often to incorporate the spices.
3. Plate and serve with avocado slices.

Tuna Imitation Salad

Nutritional Information:
Total fat: 15.8g
Cholesterol: 0mg
Sodium: 306mg
Total carbohydrates: 8.9g
Dietary fiber: 2.9g
Protein: 20.3g
Calcium: 383mg
Potassium: 54mg
Iron: 4mg
Vitamin D: 0mcg
Time: 10 minutes
Serving Size: 4
Ingredients:
- 1 block extra firm tofu, drained, pressed to remove any extra moisture and crumbled
- ¼ cup celery, finely chopped
- ¼ cup carrots, finely chopped
- 1 tsp onion powder
- 1 tsp garlic powder
- 1 tsp lemon juice
- ½ cup vegan mayonnaise
- Salt and pepper to taste

+ nutritional yeast
fresh dill
dijon

Directions:
1. Add all ingredients to a large mixing bowl and mix to combine well.
2. Chill for 15 minutes before serving. Can be served with celery sticks or other fresh cut veggies as well as used to make a sandwich. Can be stored in the refrigerator in an airtight container for up to 4 days.

Lettuce Salad Bowls

Nutritional Information:
Total fat: 17.9g
Cholesterol: 0mg
Sodium: 21mg
Total carbohydrates: 7.9g
Dietary fiber: 4.9g
Protein: 3.6g
Calcium: 72mg
Potassium: 72mg
Iron: 2mg
Vitamin D: 0mcg
Time: 10 minutes
Serving Size: 4
Ingredients:
● 1 avocado, halved, pitted and chopped
● 4 lettuce leaves
● ¼ cup purple cabbage, chopped
● 4 tbsp tahini
● Salt and pepper to taste
Directions:
1. Combine tahini and purple cabbage in a bowl. Ensure that purple cabbage is well coated.
2. To arrange salad bowls, add cabbage mixture to the center of each lettuce bowl. Top with the rest of the ingredients. Sprinkle will salt and pepper to season. Serve.

Keto Vegan Empanadas

Nutritional Information:
Total fat: 6g
Cholesterol: 0mg
Sodium: 100mg
Total carbohydrates: 15.5g
Dietary fiber: 10.7g
Protein: 2.8g
Calcium: 34mg
Potassium: 38mg
Iron: 0mg
Vitamin D: 0mcg
Time: 45 minutes
Serving Size: 8
Ingredients:

- ½ cup coconut flour
- ½ cup almond flour
- ¼ cup cold vegan butter, cubed
- ½ tsp olive oil
- ½ cup tofu, pressed, drained of any excess liquid and finely crumbled
- 1 tsp of soy sauce
- ¼ cup water
- ½ tsp paprika
- ¼ tsp ground cumin
- ¼ tsp oregano
- 2 tbsp tomato sauce
- 2 tbsp of psyllium husk
- A pinch of salt

Directions:

1. Add coconut flour, almond flour, salt vegan butter and psyllium husk to a food processor and process to form a crumbly dough. You can also do this by using your hands.
2. Add water and knead to form a wet dough. Divide the dough and form small 8 balls. Place these balls in the refrigerator to rest for up to 10 minutes.
3. To create filling, add olive oil to a small skillet and place over medium heat. Once oil is heated, add crumbled tofu. Sauté until tofu is warmed then add soy sauce, water and other spices. Stir. Bring to a boil and simmer for 5 minutes or until all the liquid has been.
4. Stir in tomato sauce and allow mixture to cool.
5. Preheat your oven to 350 degrees F.
6. Prepare a baking sheet by lining it with parchment paper.
7. Remove the dough from the refrigerator and roll out into 2 millimeter thick circles. You can also use a tortilla press to do this.
8. Place a spoonful of filling in the center of each piece of dough.
9. Fold the dough over and shape empanada. If any tears form, just smooth over gently with your fingers. Place empanada on prepared baking sheet.
10. Repeat with the rest of the dough balls.
11. Baked empanadas for 12 minutes.
12. Allow to cool slightly before serving. Can be served warm or cold. Can be served alongside a salad.

Avocado Fries

Nutritional Information:
Total fat: 15.7g
Cholesterol: 1mg
Sodium: 5mg
Total carbohydrates: 6.3g
Dietary fiber: 4.1g
Protein: 3g
Calcium: 32mg
Potassium: 297mg
Iron: 1mg
Vitamin D: 0mcg
Time: 30 minutes
Serving Size: 5
Ingredients:
- 1 large not overly ripe avocado
- 1 tsp Italian seasoning
- ¼ cup almond milk
- ½ cup almond meal

Directions:
1. Preheat your oven to 450 degrees F.
2. Prepare a baking sheet by spraying it with nonstick spray.
3. Half avocado lengthwise and pit. Peel off skin and cut into wedges of preferred size.
4. Mix the rest of the ingredients in a shallow bowl wide enough to fit avocado slices. This should form a thick batter.
5. Dip avocado slices in batter and coat thoroughly.
6. Place avocado fries on prepared baking sheet and bake for up to 20 minutes or until lightly golden.
7. Allow to cool for a few minutes then serve immediately. Can be served with your favorite keto vegan dipping sauce.

Sautéed Squash Kale Bowl

Nutritional Information:

Total fat: 18.1g

Cholesterol: 0mg

Sodium: 412mg

Total carbohydrates: 11.9g

Dietary fiber: 3.4g

Protein: 3.8g

Calcium: 69mg

Potassium: 379mg

Iron: 1mg

Vitamin D: 0mcg

Time: 30 minutes

Serving Size: 6

Ingredients:
- 2 cups butternut squash, cubed
- 2 cups kale, stems discarded, and leaves chopped
- ½ cup pecans, toasted
- 1 tsp ginger, grated
- 1 tsp garlic, grated
- 4 tbsp low-sodium tamari
- 2 tbsp olive oil

Directions:

Add olive oil to a nonstick skillet and place over medium heat. Once the oil is heated, add butternut squash. Toss to coat with oil. Cover pan and cook for 5 minutes.

Add garlic, ginger and tamari. Stir. Cook for 10 more minutes.

Add kale, cover pan and cook for 5 more minutes or until the kale leaves have wilted.

Remove pan from heat and toss in toasted pecans. Serve.

Avocado Cauliflower Salad

Nutritional Information:

Total fat: 23.1g

Cholesterol: 33mg

Sodium: 214mg

Total carbohydrates: 6.2g

Dietary fiber: 1.7g

Protein: 6.5g

Calcium:46mg

Potassium: 318mg

Iron: 1mg

Vitamin D: 0mcg

Time: 25 minutes

Serving Size: 3

Ingredients:
- 2 cups cauliflower florets
- 1/2 cup tempeh, cooked and diced
- 5 tablespoons spicy avocado mayonnaise (See recipe *Chapter 4: Sauces and Condiments: Spicy Avocado Mayonnaise*)
- 1/2 tsp fresh parsley, chopped
- Salt and pepper to taste

Directions:
1. Steam cauliflower by placing a steamer basket over a large pot with at least 2 cups of water in it. Bring water to a boil then add cauliflower florets to steamer basket. Steam cauliflower for about 8 minutes or until tender.
2. Remove cauliflower florets from heat and allow to cool down for a few minutes.
3. Add tempeh to a large skillet and crisp for about 5 minutes. Remove from heat and allow to cool completely.
4. Add all ingredients to a large bowl except for parsley and mix well to form creamy salad. Top with parsley and serve warm or chilled.

Mushroom Cauliflower Soup

Nutritional Information:
Total fat: 2.7g
Cholesterol: 0mg
Sodium: 113mg
Total carbohydrates: 10.6g
Dietary fiber: 3.5g
Protein: 2.5g
Calcium: 181mg
Potassium: 389mg
Iron: 1mg
Vitamin D: 1mcg
Time: 45 minutes
Serving Size: 3
Ingredients:
- 2 cups cauliflower florets
- 1 ½ cup white onions, diced
- 1 ½ cup unsweetened almond milk
- 1 tsp onion powder
- 1/2 tsp olive oil
- ⅓ cup mushrooms, sliced
- 2 tbsp yellow onion, diced
- Salt and pepper to taste

Directions:
1. Add cauliflower, almond milk, onion powder, salt and pepper to a saucepan and place over medium heat. Bring to a boil. Reduce heat to low and simmer for 8 minutes or until cauliflower is tender.
2. Puree mixture with an immersion blender or by adding to a food processor or blender.
3. Place another pan over high heat. Add olive oil, mushrooms and onion and sauté until onions are translucent and begin to brown slightly. This will take about 10 minutes.
4. Add pureed cauliflower mixture to sautéed mushrooms. Bring mixture to a boil, cover and simmer for 10 minutes or until sauce is thick. Serve immediately.

Zucchini Veggie Wraps

Nutritional Information:
Total fat: 6.2g
Cholesterol: 0mg
Sodium:229mg
Total carbohydrates: 5.2g
Dietary fiber: 1.8g
Protein: 2.2g
Calcium: 41mg
Potassium: 197mg
Iron: 1mg
Vitamin D: 0mcg
Time: 20 minutes
Serving Size: 10

Ingredients:
- 2 medium zucchini, thinly sliced lengthwise
- 1 yellow bell pepper, deseeded and sliced
- 1 red bell pepper, deseeded and sliced
- 6 green lettuce leaves, torn into pieces the same size as the zucchini slices
- 1 cup basil
- 1 cup spinach
- 1 garlic clove
- 2 tbsp almond butter
- 3 tbsp olive oil
- Salt and pepper to taste

Directions:
1. To create pesto dressing, add basil, spinach, garlic, almond butter, olive oil and salt to a food processor and process until a uniform consistency is achieved.
2. To assemble wraps, lay zucchini slices down first and layer with the dressing mixture.
3. Add the rest of the vegetables. Roll the zucchini and stick with a toothpick in the center. Top with salt and pepper to taste. Serve.

Cauliflower Cabbage Wraps

Nutritional Information:
Total fat: 6.5g
Cholesterol: 0mg
Sodium: 74mg
Total carbohydrates: 8.6g
Dietary fiber: 4.4g
Protein: 3.2g
Calcium: 66mg
Potassium: 333mg
Iron: 2mg
Vitamin D: 0mcg
Time: 45 minutes
Serving Size: 6
Ingredients:
- 6 green lettuce leaves
- 4 cups cauliflower florets
- 1 cup red cabbage, thinly sliced
- ½ small avocado, peeled and pitted
- 1 tbsp lime juice
- ½ tsp chili powder
- ⅓ cup cilantro, chopped
- 1 14-oz can green chilies
- ½ cup cashew butter
- 1 tbsp olive oil
- Salt and pepper to taste

Directions:
1. Preheat your oven to 400 degrees F.
2. Toss cauliflower florets with olive oil, salt and pepper and spread across a baking sheet. Roast for 30 minutes.
3. Add cashew butter, green chilies, lime juice, cilantro and chili powder in a blender and process to a smooth consistency.
4. Once the cauliflower is done roasting, toss with cashew chili sauce.
5. Mash avocado with lime juice until a creamy consistency is achieved.
6. Toss avocado mixture with red cabbage and season with salt and pepper.
7. Layer each lettuce leave with a scoop of the avocado mixture and a scoop of the cashew cauliflower mixture. Can be served with additional toppings such as hot sauce or additional cilantro.

Zucchini Green Bean Salad

Nutritional Information:
Total fat: 3.7g
Cholesterol: 1mg
Sodium: 4mg
Total carbohydrates: 8.4g
Dietary fiber: 3.2g
Protein: 2.3g
Calcium: 38mg
Potassium: 437mg
Iron: 1mg
Vitamin D: 0mcg
Time: 40 minutes
Serving Size: 9
Ingredients:
- 2 large zucchini, sliced
- 4 cups green beans, trimmed
- 2 tbsp olive oil
- 2 tsp Italian seasoning
- 4 medium tomatoes, chopped
- ½ cup fresh basil, sliced
- ½ cup balsamic vinegar
- 2 tbsp dried cranberries
- Salt and pepper to taste

Directions:
1. Preheat your grill on high heat.
2. Place green beans and zucchini in a large bowl. Whisk Italian seasoning, olive oil, salt and pepper in a small bowl. Conserve half of olive oil for dressing. Add Italian seasoning mixture to zucchini and green beans and toss so that veggies are evenly coated.
3. Place the zucchini and green beans on the grill and cook for 10 minutes or until charred. Stir occasionally.
4. To make dressing, add balsamic vinegar, cranberries, remaining olive oil, salt and pepper to a food processor and process until well mixed.
5. Add grilled veggies to a large bowl. Add chopped tomatoes. Toss with prepared balsamic vinegar dressing. Serve.

Quick and Easy Cauliflower Pizza Bites

Nutritional Information:
Total fat: 0.6g
Cholesterol: 0mg
Sodium: 31mg
Total carbohydrates: 2.5g
Dietary fiber: 1g
Protein: 0.8g
Calcium: 10mg
Potassium: 95mg
Iron: 0mg
Vitamin D: 0mcg
Time: 35 minutes
Serving Size: 12
Ingredients:

- 3 cups cauliflower florets
- ¾ cups vegan cheese, shredded
- 1 tbsp of flaxseed
- 3 tbsp water
- 3 tbsp marinara sauce
- ½ tsp garlic powder
- ½ tsp onion powder
- Salt and pepper to taste

Directions:

1. Preheat your oven to 400 degrees F.
2. Prepare a 12 mini muffin tin pan by lining with parchment paper strips.
3. Add cauliflower to food processor and process until a rice like consistency is achieved.
4. Transfer cauliflower rice to microwave-safe bowl. Microwave for 5 minutes.
5. Allow cauliflower to cool for a few minutes then place in a cheesecloth and squeeze tightly to remove any excess moisture.
6. Add cauliflower to a large mixing bowl. Add all the other ingredients to the mixing bowl and mix. Reserve 1/4 cup of vegan cheese.
7. Scoop out tablespoonfuls of cauliflower mixture and place in cups of muffin tin pan.
8. Press the mixture down tightly and bake for 15 minutes.
9. Remove the pizza bites from the oven and top with remaining vegan cheese then broil for 1 minute.
10. Allow the cauliflower pizza bites to cool down for 15 minutes then remove from pan by pulling on the parchment paper edges. Can be served with marinara sauce.

Chapter 7: Dinner Recipes

Breakfast gives you nutrition to kick-start the day and lunch is the great opportunity to refuel and refocus to keep that same energy throughout the rest of the day. This begs the question of why dinner is important. The first reason is that this meal provides fuel for the body so that you do not wake up in the middle of the night hungry. This interruption can disrupt your sleep patterns, make you gain inadequate amounts of sleep, and cause you to feel drained the next day. Eating dinner is also the perfect opportunity to spend time with your family and friends which helps with social bonding.

There is a common misperception that skipping dinner results in weight loss but, more often than not, the opposite is true. Not eating dinner can actually make it more difficult to lose weight because the body goes into survival mode when it is starved and stores more fat.

It is essential that you partake in this meal so here are a few tips to ensure that you get the best out of your dinner:

● Eat slowly and relax so that your body can properly digest the nutrition that you are providing. Eating slowly also helps in weight loss management since it takes the body about 20 minutes to register that it is full. Eating slowly allows you to not overeat.
● Eat early in the evening so that your body has an adequate amount of time to digest a meal before bedtime. This helps reduce the risk of developing obesity and weight loss problems, helps lower the risk of developing cancer, helps improve heart health, improves energy and mood levels, improves digestive health and helps you sleep better.
● Do not partake in foods that are high in carbohydrates as they increase blood sugar and make it difficult to fall asleep and stay asleep during the night.

After realizing how important the last meal of the day is, I am sure that you are eager to get started in trying out the recipes outlined below.

Cauliflower Steaks

Nutritional Information:
Total fat: 3g
Cholesterol: 0mg
Sodium: 283mg
Total carbohydrates: 9.4g
Dietary fiber: 4.3g
Protein: 3.4g
Calcium: 39mg
Potassium: 517mg
Iron: 1mg
Vitamin D: 0mcg
Time: 45 minutes
Serving Size: 5
Ingredients:
- 1 large head cauliflower
- 1 tbsp olive oil
- ½ tsp curry powder
- 1 garlic clove, grated
- 1 tbsp lime juice
- ½ teaspoon salt

Directions:
1. Thoroughly washed the cauliflower and allow to dry. Trim of the leaves and the bottom stem off the cauliflower. Leave the core intact and cut through the center of the cauliflower to ensure that the florets remain intact. Cut one inch slices and place in a large mixing bowl.
2. In a small bowl, create the marinade by combining the rest of the ingredients. Pour over cauliflower steaks, mix and allow to sit for 1 hour.
3. Preheat your oven to 400 degrees F.
4. Prepare a baking sheet by lining it with parchment paper.
5. Place marinated cauliflower steaks on the prepared baking sheet and bake for 20 minutes or until cauliflower is crisp at the edges. Serve with a side of roasted veggies.

Veggie Walnut Soup

Nutritional Information:
Total fat: 17.1g
Cholesterol: 0mg
Sodium: 34mg
Total carbohydrates: 11.7g
Dietary fiber: 4.1g
Protein: 6.8g
Calcium: 56mg
Potassium: 640mg
Iron: 2mg
Vitamin D: 0mcg
Time: 45 minutes
Serving Size: 8
Ingredients:
- 5 celery stalks, finely diced
- 2 green bell peppers, finely diced
- 2 medium zucchini, diced
- 8 oz cremini mushrooms
- 1 cup raw walnuts, minced
- 2 garlic cloves, minced
- 2 tbsp olive oil
- 1 tsp ground cinnamon
- 2 tsp chili powder
- 4 tsp ground cumin
- 1 tsp smoked paprika
- 1 tbsp tomato paste
- ½ cup coconut milk
- 3 cups water
- 1 tbsp unsweetened cocoa powder
- 2 cup tomatoes, diced
- Salt and pepper to taste

Directions:
1. Over medium heat, heat olive oil in a large pot. Add celery and sauté for 4 minutes.
2. Add cumin, paprika, chili powder, cinnamon and garlic and sauté until mixture becomes fragrant or about 2 minutes.
3. Add mushrooms, zucchini, and bell peppers and sauté for 5 more minutes.
4. Add tomato paste, tomatoes, coconut milk, water, walnuts and cocoa powder. Reduce heat to low and simmer for 25 minutes or until the sauce thickens and vegetables are so soft.
5. Season with salt and pepper and serve.

Roasted Red Pepper Soup

Nutritional Information:
Total fat: 17.1g
Cholesterol: 0mg
Sodium: 552mg
Total carbohydrates: 9.6g
Dietary fiber: 4g
Protein: 3.4g
Calcium: 41mg
Potassium: 482mg
Iron: 1mg
Vitamin D: 0mcg
Time: 30 minutes
Serving Size: 5
Ingredients:
- ½ cup roasted red peppers, chopped
- 5 cups cauliflower florets
- 4 cups water
- ½ tsp apple cider vinegar
- 1 cup coconut milk
- 2 tbsp coconut oil
- 1 scallion, finely chopped
- 1 tsp salt
- 1 tsp smoked paprika
- A pinch of red pepper flakes, crushed
- A pinch of fresh thyme

Directions:
1. Add coconut oil to a heavy-bottomed pan and place over medium heat. Add scallions and sauté for 3 minutes.
2. Add roasted red peppers and all spices and sauté for 3 minutes.
3. Add cauliflower water and vinegar. Bring to a simmer, cover pot and allow to cook for 15 minutes or until the cauliflower is soft and breaking apart easily.
4. Use an immersion blender to blend to a smooth consistency.
5. Add coconut milk and cook until warm. Serve.

Zucchini Spinach Ravioli

Nutritional Information:
Total fat: 23.7g
Cholesterol: 0mg
Sodium: 461mg
Total carbohydrates: 12.8g
Dietary fiber: 3.8g
Protein: 11.1g
Calcium: 51mg
Potassium: 499mg
Iron: 3mg
Vitamin D: 0mcg
Time: 1 hour
Serving Size: 7
Ingredients:
- 4 medium zucchini, sliced with mandolin
- 1 cup fresh spinach
- 1 cup raw cashews
- 1 cup walnuts
- 1 cup water
- 1 cup fresh basil
- 1 ½ tsp salt
- ½ tsp ground black pepper
- ¼ cup pine nuts
- 4 garlic cloves
- ¼ cup hemp hearts
- Cashew Cheese Sauce (See Recipes *Chapter 4: Sauces and Condiments: Keto Vegan Raw Cashew Cheese Sauce*)

Directions:
1. Preheat your oven to 350 degrees F.
2. Prepare a baking sheet by lining it with parchment paper.
3. Place zucchini slices on paper towels and sprinkle with salt to draw out excess moisture. Allow to sit.
4. Create "Parmesan" by placing pine nuts, hemp hearts and salt in a food processor and pulse to a crumbly texture. Set aside
5. Place spinach, cashews, walnuts, garlic, salt, pepper, water and basil in a food processor and pulse to a ricotta-like texture.
6. Wipe off any remaining moisture from zucchini slices and taking 4 at a time, make an X shape. Place a spoonful of ricotta mixture and place in the center where the zucchini slices meet.
7. Fold the tips of the zucchini over to make a ravioli pocket. Place in the prepared baking sheet and repeat until all the zucchini slices have been used up. Make enough ravioli for a serving of 4 each.
8. Sprinkle with Parmesan mixture.
9. Bake for 30 minutes or until zucchini is fully cooked.
10. Allow to sit for 15 minutes before serving. Top with cashew cheese sauce and serve.

Keto Vegan Shepherd's Pie

Nutritional Information:
Total fat: 7.4g
Cholesterol: 0mg
Sodium: 47mg
Total carbohydrates: 14.5g
Dietary fiber: 3.9g
Protein: 7.1g
Calcium: 68mg
Potassium: 455mg
Iron: 3mg
Vitamin D: 41mcg
Time: 1 hour 10 minutes
Serving Size: 8
Ingredients:
- 6 cups cauliflower florets
- 1 yellow onion, diced
- 2 medium carrots, peeled and diced
- 3 garlic cloves, chopped
- 1 celery stalk, diced
- 5 dried wild mushrooms
- 3 cups cremini mushrooms, diced
- ¼ cup water
- 1 cup vegetable stock
- 4 tbsp olive oil
- 1 tbsp thyme leaves, roughly chopped
- 1 tbsp tomato paste
- 3 tbsp nutritional yeast
- A pinch ground nutmeg

Directions:
1. Reconstitute wild mushrooms by soaking in 1/4 cup boiling water for 30 minutes.
2. Preheat your oven to 400 degrees F.
3. Prepare a baking pan by greasing it with vegan butter or extra olive oil.
4. Add cauliflower florets to a large saucepan. Cover with water, add salt and place pan over medium heat. Bring to a boil and cook cauliflower until tender. Drain and set aside.
5. Place a large frying pan over medium heat and add 2 tablespoons of olive oil, carrots, onion, and celery. Cook until the vegetables become caramelized.
6. Add the cremini mushrooms in increments of 4. Ensure that each increment is cooked before adding the next.
7. Remove the wild mushrooms from the water. Reserve water. Roughly chop the mushrooms. Add to the frying pan.
8. Increase the heat from medium to high and add tomato paste and 1/4 cup of water. Cook until the liquid has almost evaporated before adding the wild mushrooms, liquid reserved from soaking the mushrooms, and vegetable stock.
9. Reduce heat to low and simmer for 10 minutes or until half of the liquid has evaporated. Remove the pan from the heat.
10. Add cauliflower to a food processor along with 2 tablespoons of olive oil, nutritional yeast, thyme leaves, nutmeg and salt. Blend until a smooth creamy consistency is achieved.

11. Pour mushroom mixture into the bottom of the prepared baking pan. Spread evenly on the bottom of the pan.
12. Top with the cauliflower mash. Smooth the top with a spatula.
13. Bake for 20 minutes or until the top is golden brown.
14. Allow to cool completely before dividing into serving plates.

Green Soup

Nutritional Information:
Total fat: 0.3g
Cholesterol: 0mg
Sodium: 200mg
Total carbohydrates: 11g
Dietary fiber: 3.6g
Protein: 3.6g
Calcium: 83mg
Potassium: 483mg
Iron: 2mg
Vitamin D: 0mcg
Time: 45 minutes
Serving Size: 6
Ingredients:
- 3 cups cauliflower, chopped
- 3 cups broccoli, chopped
- 1 large leek, chopped
- 3 cups water
- 2 cups kale
- 1 tbsp soy sauce
- ½ cup parsley
- 1 sprig of thyme
- 1 tsp turmeric
- 2 bay leaves
- 1 teaspoon garlic powder

Directions:
1. Cover chopped cauliflower and broccoli with water in a large pot and boil for 10 minutes over medium-high heat until just tender.
2. Add remaining ingredients and simmer for 10 minutes or until the kale is cooked.
3. Remove bay leaves and add mixture to blender. Blend until a smooth creamy consistency is achieved.
4. Divide into serving bowls and serve. Can be topped with roasted veggies.

Portobello Mushroom Tacos with Guacamole

Nutritional Information:
Total fat: 18.7g
Cholesterol: 3mg
Sodium: 131mg
Total carbohydrates: 12g
Dietary fiber: 4.9g
Protein: 4.4g
Calcium: 24mg
Potassium: 566mg
Iron: 1mg
Vitamin D: 0mcg
Time: 35 minutes
Serving Size: 7
Ingredients:
- 1 lb. portobello mushrooms, destemmed, rinsed and dried
- 3 tbsp olive oil
- 1 tsp ground cumin
- 1 tsp onion powder
- 1/4 cup harissa
- 7 lettuce leaves, rinsed and dried
- 2 ripe medium avocados
- 2 tbsp tomatoes, chopped
- 2 tbsp red onion, chopped
- 2 tbsp lime juice
- 1 tbsp cilantro, chopped
- A pinch of salt

Directions:
1. Mix half of olive oil, cumin, onion powder and harissa in a small bowl.
2. Brush each mushroom with cumin mixture, ensuring well coated. Allow to marinade for at least 15 minutes.
3. Prepare guacamole while mushrooms are marinating by halving and pitting avocados and scooping out the flesh. Add avocados, chopped tomatoes, red onions, lime juice, salt and cilantro to a bowl and mash to desired consistency.
4. When the mushrooms are done marinating, heat the remaining olive oil in a non-stick skillet over medium high. When the oil has become heated, place the mushrooms in the pan and cook for 3 minutes or until edges are browned. Flip and cook for another 3 minutes.
5. Turn off the heat and allow the mushrooms to rest for 3 minutes before slicing.
6. Fill each lettuce leaf with a few slices of portobello. Add guacamole and other desired toppings like more chopped tomatoes and cilantro. Serve.

Roasted Mushroom Burgers

Nutritional Information:
Total fat: 9.1g
Cholesterol: 5mg
Sodium: 316mg
Total carbohydrates: 6.5g
Dietary fiber: 2.9g
Protein: 6.5g
Calcium: 90mg
Potassium: 248mg
Iron: 3mg
Vitamin D: 189mcg
Time: 45 minutes
Serving Size: 4
Ingredients:
- 3 cups mushrooms, cooked and chopped
- 1 tbsp chia seeds
- ½ tsp salt
- ¼ tsp black pepper
- 3 tbsp protein powder
- ¼ tsp sweet paprika
- ¼ cup tahini

Directions:
1. Preheat your oven to 350 degrees F.
2. Prepare a baking sheet by lining it with parchment paper.
3. Add chopped mushrooms to food processor and pulse to a coarse consistency.
4. Transfer mushrooms to a mixing bowl and stir in chia seeds, salt, pepper, rosemary and tahini. Combine thoroughly. Allow mixture to stand for 5 minutes so that it thickens.
5. Stir in protein powder gradually until completely absorbed. If the protein powder stops being easily incorporated, stop adding protein powder so that the mixture does not become dry.
6. Form equally-sized patties and place them on the prepared baking sheet.
7. Bake for 25 minutes or until patties are firm.
8. Remove patties from oven and allow to cool for a few minutes before serving your favorite keto vegan bread topped with veggies and keto vegan friendly sauce.

Roasted Radishes

Nutritional Information:
Total fat: 5g
Cholesterol: 0mg
Sodium: 281mg
Total carbohydrates: 2g
Dietary fiber: 0.8g
Protein: 0.9g
Calcium: 28mg
Potassium: 88mg
Iron: 1mg
Vitamin D: 0mcg
Time: 30 minutes
Serving Size: 5
Ingredients:
- 25 medium radishes, washed, trimmed and quartered
- 2 green onions, sliced
- 1 ½ tbsp soy sauce
- 1 ½ tbsp peanut oil
- 3 tsp sesame seeds

Directions:
1. Preheat your oven to 425 degrees F.
2. Prepare a baking sheet by spraying it with nonstick spray.
3. Place the radishes on the baking sheet and brush with peanut oil. Arrange radishes cut side down so that it browns in the best manner.
4. Roast radishes for 20 minutes, stirring halfway through.
5. Mixed together soy sauce and any remaining peanut oil.
6. Remove radishes from the oven at the 20 minute mark and brush with the soy sauce mixture. Sprinkle with green onions. Bake for 5 more minutes.
7. Toast sesame seeds by placing in a hot dry pan and shaking pan for 1 minute over medium heat.
8. Sprinkle roasted radishes with toasted sesame seeds and serve hot. Can be served with your favorite keto vegan dipping sauce.

Roasted Pepper Zoodles

Nutritional Information:
Total fat: 16.8g
Cholesterol: 0mg
Sodium: 25mg
Total carbohydrates: 10.3g
Dietary fiber: 3.3g
Protein: 4.4g
Calcium: 27mg
Potassium: 428mg
Iron: 2mg
Vitamin D: 0mcg
Time: 25 minutes
Serving Size: 6
Ingredients:
- 2 red bell peppers, sliced
- ½ cup fresh arugula
- ½ cup fresh basil
- ¼ cup fresh cilantro
- 5 tbsp olive oil
- ¼ cup nutritional yeast
- 2 medium zucchini, spiralized into noodles
- 1 tbsp vegan butter
- 2 garlic cloves, minced
- 2 tsp lemon juice
- Salt and pepper to taste

Directions:
1. Preheat your oven to 300 degrees F.
2. Prepare a baking sheet by spraying it with nonstick spray. Place pepper slices skin side up in a single layer on prepared baking sheet. Place in oven broiler and broil for 10 minutes or until pepper skin chars.
3. Place peppers in food processor. Add arugula, basil, nutritional yeast, cilantro, salt and pepper. Process while streaming in 3 tablespoons of olive oil.
4. Place the rest of olive oil and vegan butter into a large skillet. Place over medium heat. Add garlic once the oil has heated and cook for 1 minute.
5. Add lemon juice and zucchini noodles and cook for 5 minutes or until the noodles soften slightly. Toss often.
6. Add pepper mixture and cook for 5 minutes.
7. Serve. Can be topped with nutritional yeast for a cheesier flavor.

Creamy Curry Zucchini Noodles

Nutritional Information:
Total fat: 16.5g
Cholesterol: 16mg
Sodium: 585mg
Total carbohydrates: 10g
Dietary fiber: 3.5g
Protein: 2.9g
Calcium: 42mg
Potassium: 569mg
Iron: 2mg
Vitamin D: 0mcg
Time: 20 minutes
Serving Size: 5
Ingredients:
- 2 large zucchini, spiralized
- 2 tbsp olive oil
- 2 cups cauliflower florets
- 1 red bell pepper, diced
- ¼ cup cilantro, chopped
- ¼ cup avocado mayonnaise (See recipe *Chapter 4: Sauces and Condiments: Spicy Avocado Mayonnaise*)
- 2 tbsp avocado oil
- 1 tsp ground ginger
- ½ tsp ground black pepper
- 1 tsp salt
- 1 tsp ground turmeric
- 1 tsp ground cumin
- 2 tsp curry powder
- 2 tbsp apple cider vinegar
- ¼ cup water

Directions:
1. Add olive oil to a large nonstick skillet and place over medium heat. Once the oil is hot, sauté zucchini noodles for 5 minutes, stirring occasionally.
2. Remove from heat and allowed to cool for 10 minutes.
3. Transfer zucchini noodles to a large mixing bowl. Add cauliflower, bell peppers and cilantro. Mix well.
4. To make creamy curry sauce, add the rest of the ingredients to a blender and blend until a smooth and creamy consistency is achieved.
5. Pour creamy curry sauce over zucchini and vegetable mixture and toss to coat.
6. Serve immediately or place in the refrigerator to chill for a few hours. Can be stored in an airtight container in the refrigerator for up to 2 days.

Creamy Spinach Shirataki

Nutritional Information:
Total fat: 6.9g
Cholesterol: 0mg
Sodium: 143mg
Total carbohydrates: 7.9g
Dietary fiber: 0.9g
Protein: 1.5g
Calcium: 23mg
Potassium: 60mg
Iron: 0mg
Vitamin D: 0mcg
Time: 25 minutes
Serving Size: 6
Ingredients:
- 1 package Shirataki noodles, drained and rinsed
- 2 oz vegan cream cheese
- 1 cup fresh spinach
- 1 yellow onion, chopped
- 1 tbsp olive oil
- 1 tsp garlic powder
- ½ cup full fat coconut milk
- Salt and pepper to taste

Directions:
1. Salt and pepper to taste
2. Add oil to a nonstick skillet and place over medium heat. When the heat oil is heated, add onions and sauté until onions are translucent.
3. Add spinach and sauté until leaves are wilted.
4. Add all the other ingredients and cook until liquid reduces, and a creamy texture is achieved. Serve.

Tempeh Broccoli Stir Fry Dinner

Nutritional Information:
Total fat: 5.9g
Cholesterol: 0mg
Sodium: 16mg
Total carbohydrates: 4.3g
Dietary fiber: 0.8g
Protein: 4.9g
Calcium: 42mg
Potassium: 210mg
Iron: 1mg
Vitamin D: 0mcg
Time: 25 minutes
Serving Size: 4
Ingredients:
- 3 oz tempeh, chopped
- 1 cup broccoli florets
- 1 cup frozen spinach
- 1 tbsp olive oil
- 1 tsp garlic powder
- Salt and pepper to taste
- Fresh chopped cilantro to garnish

Directions:
1. Add olive oil to a nonstick skillet and place over medium heat. Once the oil has become heated, add tempeh pieces and sauté for about 5 minutes or until the pieces begin to brown. Stir frequently.
2. Add the rest of the ingredients and sauté for about 2 more minutes or until spinach leaves have wilted. Stir occasionally.
3. Divide between serving plates and garnish. Serve.

Sautéed Brussel Sprouts Dish

Nutritional Information:
Total fat: 3.5g
Cholesterol: 0mg
Sodium: 109mg
Total carbohydrates: 9.2g
Dietary fiber: 3.4g
Protein: 4g
Calcium: 48mg
Potassium: 324mg
Iron: 1mg
Vitamin D: 0mcg
Time: 20 minutes
Serving Size: 2
Ingredients:

- 1 cup of Brussel sprouts, chopped
- ½ tsp olive oil
- 1 garlic clove, minced
- 1 tsp onion powder
- 1 cup frozen spinach
- Salt and pepper to taste
- 3 tbsp cauliflower hummus (See recipe *Chapter 4: Sauces and Condiments: Cauliflower Hummus*)

Directions:

1. Add olive oil to a skillet and place over medium heat to heat oil. Once oil is hot, add the Brussel sprouts and garlic and shake the pan so that all the cut sides of the Brussel sprouts settle down in a single layer in the pan.
2. Sauté undisturbed for 5 minutes the cut sides of the sprouts begin to caramelize.
3. Stir, add spinach and cook for 6 more minutes.
4. Add the rest of the ingredients. Stir and cook for 1 more minute.
5. Plate. Top with cauliflower hummus and serve.

Cauliflower Pizza Crust with Veggie Toppings

Nutritional Information:
Total fat: 7.2g
Cholesterol: 0mg
Sodium: 178mg
Total carbohydrates: 7.6g
Dietary fiber: 3.5g
Protein: 3.6g
Calcium: 51mg
Potassium: 50mg
Iron: 1mg
Vitamin D: 0mcg
Time: 1 hour
Serving Size: 5
Ingredients:
- 2 cups cauliflower rice, cooked
- ¼ cup tahini
- ¼ tsp salt
- ¼ cup whole psyllium husk

Directions:
1. Preheat your oven to 375 degrees F.
2. Prepare a baking sheet by lining it with parchment paper.
3. Mix all ingredients to form a uniform dough.
4. Roll the dough out into a 1/4 inch thick circle and place on the prepared baking sheet.
5. Bake for 15 minutes. Flip over and bake for an additional 10 minutes or until crust is golden brown.
6. Remove the dough from the oven and top with your favorite savory keto vegan sauce and fresh, sautéed or roasted veggies. Serve.

Tofu Tomato Stir Fry

Nutritional Information:
Total fat: 7.9g
Cholesterol: 0mg
Sodium: 336mg
Total carbohydrates: 5.5g
Dietary fiber: 1.1g
Protein: 3.1g
Calcium: 40mg
Potassium: 182mg
Iron: 1mg
Vitamin D: 0mcg
Time: 10 minutes
Serving Size: 2
Ingredients:
- ½ cup tomato, sliced
- ¼ block firm tofu
- 1 tbsp sesame oil
- 1 tbsp low-sodium tamari
- ½ cup cauliflower rice, cooked
- 2 green onions, sliced
- Salt and pepper to taste

Directions:
1. Add sesame oil and tamari to non-stick skillet and place over medium heat. Once oil heated, add green onions and sliced tomato. Toss then cover pan with lid and allow to cook for 5 minutes or until the tomatoes are soft.
2. Add tofu to pan and crumble with a fork. Stir so that the tofu is coated with the oil mixture. Cook for 2 minutes with the pan uncovered to allow the tofu to become warmed. This will allow the excess liquid to evaporate.
3. Remove the pan from the heat and seasoned with salt and pepper. Serve over cauliflower rice.

Walnut Zucchini Chili

Nutritional Information:
Total fat: 19.7g
Cholesterol: 0mg
Sodium: 58mg
Total carbohydrates: 15.1g
Dietary fiber: 5.3g
Protein: 12.5g
Calcium: 180mg
Potassium: 812mg
Iron: 3mg
Vitamin D: 0mcg
Time: 50 minutes
Serving Size: 8
Ingredients:
- 2 medium zucchini, diced
- 1 cup raw walnuts, minced
- 2 yellow bell peppers, finely diced
- 8 oz cremini mushrooms
- 4 celery stalks, finely diced
- 1 yellow onion, diced
- 2 garlic cloves, minced
- 1 tsp ground cinnamon
- 2 tsp chili powder
- 3 tsp ground cumin
- 1 tsp smoked paprika
- 1 tbsp tomato paste
- 2 large tomatoes, diced
- 1 tbsp unsweetened cocoa powder
- ½ cup coconut milk
- 3 cups water
- 2 tbsp olive oil
- 2 cups tofu, crumbled

Directions:
1. Add olive oil to a large pot and place over medium heat. Add celery and onion and cook for 4 minutes or until onion is translucent.
2. Add cinnamon, chili powder, cumin, paprika and garlic and sauté for 2 more minutes or until fragrant.
3. Add bell peppers, mushrooms and zucchini and cook for 5 more minutes.
4. Add tomato paste, tomatoes, coconut milk, tofu, water, walnuts and cocoa powder. Reduce heat to low and simmer for 25 minutes or until the sauce is thick and vegetables are soft.
5. Season with salt and pepper to taste. Serve.

Roasted Veggies on Broccoli Rice

Nutritional Information:
Total fat: 23.2g
Cholesterol: 0mg
Sodium: 117mg
Total carbohydrates: 16.9g
Dietary fiber: 6.7g
Protein: 6.5g
Calcium: 60mg
Potassium: 796mg
Iron: 3mg
Vitamin D: 0mcg
Time: 1 hour
Serving Size: 7
Ingredients:
- 1 head of broccoli
- 2 red bell peppers, chopped
- 2 cups cauliflower florets
- ⅓ cup olive oil
- 6 sun-dried tomatoes, chopped
- 1/2 cup pitted black olives
- 1 large avocado, sliced
- ¼ cup pumpkin seeds
- ¼ cup pine nuts
- ¼ cup sunflower seeds
- ¼ cup fresh parsley, finely chopped
- 1 tbsp fresh chives, finely chopped
- 1 tbsp fresh mint, finely chopped
- 1 tbsp nutritional yeast
- 1 tbsp coconut aminos
- ½ tbsp lime juice
- Salt and pepper to taste

Directions:
1. Preheat oven to 400 degrees F.
2. Placed chopped peppers and cauliflower florets on a baking sheet. Toss with 1 tablespoon of olive oil and a pinch of salt. Roast for 40 minutes or until veggies are soft.
3. While vegetables roast, add broccoli florets to a food processor and pulse until a rice like consistency is achieved.
4. Place all seeds and pine nuts on a baking tray. Toss with a pinch of salt and a small amount of olive oil. Roast for 5 minutes or until golden brown.
5. To make dressing, add remaining olive oil, coconut aminos, lime juice and a pinch of salt and pepper to a small bowl and whisk.
6. Fluff broccoli rice then add dressing, seeds, nuts, roasted veggies, sun-dried tomatoes, olives, avocado, herbs and nutritional yeast, and toss. Serve.

Keto Vegan Thai Curry

Nutritional Information:
Total fat: 14.6g
Cholesterol: 0mg
Sodium: 813mg
Total carbohydrates: 9.5g
Dietary fiber: 1.5g
Protein: 4.5g
Calcium: 50mg
Potassium: 255mg
Iron: 2mg
Vitamin D: 0mcg
Time: 25 minutes
Serving Size: 5
Ingredients:
- 1 block tofu, cubed
- 1 tsp Thai curry paste
- 2 tbsp coconut oil
- 1 tbsp peanut butter
- 1 tbsp tomato paste
- 2 ½ cup full fat coconut milk
- 2 tsp chili flakes
- 1 tsp ginger, grated
- 1 garlic clove, minced
- ¼ cup soy sauce
- 2 red bell peppers, cut into strips
- 1 stalk lemongrass, chopped

Directions:
1. Add coconut oil to a nonstick pan and place over medium heat. Add ginger and garlic and stir.
2. Add bell peppers and lemongrass. Stir for about 30 seconds then add coconut milk and chili flakes. Stir for 30 more seconds
3. Add the rest of the ingredients except for tofu cubes. Stir for 1 minute.
4. Add tofu cubes and allow curry cook for 10 minutes or until the sauce thickens.
5. Divide curry into serving bowls and serve.

Falafel with Tahini Sauce

Nutritional Information:
Total fat: 7.8g
Cholesterol: 0mg
Sodium: 299mg
Total carbohydrates: 7.1g
Dietary fiber: 4.1g
Protein: 2.9g
Calcium: 30mg
Potassium: 137mg
Iron: 1mg
Vitamin D: 0mcg
Time: 30 minutes
Serving Size: 8
Ingredients:
- 1 ½ cup cauliflower florets
- 2 tbsp olive oil
- 2 tbsp flax seeds
- 6 tablespoons water
- ½ cup slivered almonds
- 1 garlic clove, minced
- 2 tbsp fresh parsley, chopped
- 3 tbsp coconut flour
- 1 tbsp ground cumin
- 1/2 tbsp ground coriander
- 1 tsp salt
- ½ tsp cayenne pepper

Directions:
1. Create egg substitute by combining flaxseed and water in a small bowl. Set aside for 5 minutes.
2. Add cauliflower to a food processor and pulse until a grainy texture is achieved.
3. Add almonds to a food processor and pulse to a crumbly texture.
4. Combine cauliflower and almonds in a medium mixing bowl. Add the rest of the ingredients except for olive oil and stir to combine well.
5. Form 3 inch wide patties with the mixture. Press down until the patties are about 1/2 inch thick.
6. Add olive oil to a nonstick skillet and place over medium heat. When the oil is sizzling and add the panties and fry for 5 minutes or until the bottom edge browns.
7. Flip and fry for 5 more minutes. Remove patties and place on a paper towel lined plate to drain excess oil. Serve with tahini sauce or any other favorite keto vegan dipping sauce.

Chapter 8: Dessert and Snacks Recipes

Snacking is not the terrible villain it is made out to be. Not when it is done in the right way. In fact, snacking has a variety of benefits that include:
- Improving overall health
- Curbing cravings
- Regulating mood
- Boosting brain power
- Lowering the risk of developing heart disease
- Managing weight gain
- Providing energy throughout the day
- Help injects diet with nutrition that might have been missed during main meals

Snacking has gotten such a bad rap because most people reach for an unhealthy items such as those filled with sugar and unhealthy fats instead of healthy alternatives such as fruits and veggies. Not only do these contribute to negative health effects it also leads to overeating which can lead to excessive weight gain and even obesity.

The best way to avoid these negative consequences is to have healthy snacks on hand so that you can curb your cravings, eat smaller amounts, lower your blood sugar and keep your metabolism revved throughout the day. Below are 15 healthy keto vegan snack and dessert recipes you can keep on hand and indulge in when hunger strikes. Remember that moderation and careful planning are the keys to healthy snacking.

Baked Zucchini Chips

Nutritional Information:
Total fat: 1.5g
Cholesterol: 0mg
Sodium: 120mg
Total carbohydrates: 1.3g
Dietary fiber: 0.4g
Protein: 0.5g
Calcium: 6mg
Potassium: 103mg
Iron: 0mg
Vitamin D: 0mcg
Time: 2 hours 45 minutes
Serving Size: 10
Ingredients:
- 2 medium zucchini, sliced with a mandolin
- 1 tbsp olive oil
- 1/2 tsp salt

Directions:
1. Preheat your oven to 200 degrees F.
2. Prepare your baking sheets by lining with parchment paper.
3. Add all ingredients to a large mixing bowl and toss to thoroughly coat the zucchini with oil and salt.
4. Arrange the zucchini slices in a single layer on the baking sheet. They can touch but they should not overlap.
5. Bake for 2 and a half hours or until the zucchini chips are golden and crispy.
6. Turn off the oven and allow them to cool with the oven door cropped slightly open. This will allow the zucchini chips to crisp up even more as they cool.

Gluten-Free Nut-Free Red Velvet Cupcakes

Nutritional Information:
Total fat: 2.9g
Cholesterol: 0mg
Sodium: 93mg
Total carbohydrates: 4.9g
Dietary fiber: 2.4g
Protein: 1.8g
Calcium: 53mg
Potassium: 196mg
Iron: 2mg
Vitamin D: 0mcg
Time: 50 minutes
Serving Size: 8
Ingredients:
- 2 tbsp flax meal
- 4 tbsp cocoa powder
- ½ cup of almond butter
- ½ cup unsweetened almond milk
- 1 tbsp granulated erythritol
- 2 tbsp apple cider vinegar
- 4 tbsp ground flaxseed
- 1 tsp baking powder
- 1/2 tsp baking soda

Directions:
1. Preheat your oven to 350 degrees F.
2. Prepare a standard size muffin tin by lining it with paper liners.
3. In a small bowl, whisk together almond butter, almond milk and apple cider vinegar until a smooth combined mixture is achieved. Stir in flax seeds and erythritol and set aside.
4. In a large mixing bowl, sift together cocoa powder, flax meal, baking powder and baking soda. Mix to combine.
5. Pour the wet mixture into the dry ingredients and stir until there are no lumps. Do not overmix.
6. Divide the batter between the lined muffin wells. Ensure that each muffin is filled 3/4 of the way. Bake for 30 minutes or until the top of each muffin is firm to the touch.
7. Remove from the oven and allow to cool in pan for 10 minutes. Remove the cupcakes from the pan and allow to cool completely. Serve.

5-Ingredient Ice-cream

Nutritional Information:
Total fat: 10.1g
Cholesterol: 0mg
Sodium: 34mg
Total carbohydrates: 3.7
Dietary fiber: 0.9g
Protein: 4.7g
Calcium: 1mg
Potassium: 6mg
Iron: 2mg
Vitamin D: 0mcg
Time: 1 hour 10 minutes
Serving Size: 6
Ingredients:
- 1 ½ cup full fat coconut milk
- ⅓ cup natural peanut butter
- 2 tbsp vanilla extract
- ⅛ tsp stevia powder
- A pinch of salt

Directions:
1. Prior to starting this recipe, place a freezer-safe container in the freezer for at least 24 hours before to ensure that when the ice cream mixture is transferred no ice crystals are formed.
2. Add all ingredients to a blender and blend until a smooth and creamy consistency is achieved.
3. Chill this mixture by placing it in the refrigerator for 1 hour.
4. Transfer the mixture to an ice-cream maker and churn for 10 minutes or until it achieves a soft serve consistency.
5. Transfer the ice cream to the prepared freezer-safe container and freeze for at least one hour before serving. Can be served with caramel sauce (See recipe *Chapter 4: Sauces and Condiments: Keto Caramel Sauce*)

Peanut Butter Cups

Nutritional Information:
Total fat: 5.7g
Cholesterol: 0mg
Sodium: 33mg
Total carbohydrates: 3.2g
Dietary fiber: 0.9g
Protein: 2g
Calcium: 0mg
Potassium: 47mg
Iron: 1mg
Vitamin D: 0mcg
Time: 45 minutes
Serving Size: 18
Ingredients:
- ½ cup peanut butter
- 1 cup sugar-free dark chocolate chips
- 1 tbsp coconut oil

Directions:
1. Place the chocolate chips and coconut oil in a microwave-safe bowl. Microwave in 15 second bursts to melt the chocolate. Stir to combine the two ingredients.
2. Put a spoonful of chocolate into foil candy cups. Swirl so that the chocolate coats the sides of the cups. Pour excess chocolate back into the bowl.
3. Place the chocolate lined cups in the freezer for 10 minutes or until chocolate is set.
4. While the chocolate is setting, place the peanut butter in a microwave-safe bowl and microwave in 15 second bursts until the peanut butter becomes pourable.
5. Pour a spoonful of peanut butter into each of the chocolate-set cups. Tap the cups on a flat surface to smooth the tops of the peanut butter.
6. Pour a spoonful of melted chocolate on top of the peanut butter in each cup.
7. Place in the freezer for 10 minutes to set chocolate. Unmold and serve. Can be stored in the refrigerator in an airtight container for up to 3 days or in the freezer for up to 1 month.

Chocolate Avocado Mousse

Nutritional Information:
Total fat: 16.2g
Cholesterol:0mg
Sodium: 62mg
Total carbohydrates: 14.1g
Dietary fiber: 5.3g
Protein: 2.5g
Calcium: 24mg
Potassium: 402mg
Iron: 1mg
Vitamin D: 0mcg
Time: 10 minutes
Serving Size: 6
Ingredients:
- ½ cup dark chocolate chips
- 3 tbsp cocoa powder
- 2 large ripe avocados
- ¼ cup unsweetened almond milk
- 1 tsp vanilla extract
- ⅛ tsp salt
- Strawberries for topping

Directions:
1. Place chocolate chips in a microwave-safe bowl and microwave in 15 second bursts until the chocolate is melted but not burnt. Stir and set aside. Let cool until just barely warm.
2. Remove the pits from the avocados and scoop out the flesh. Place the flesh into a food processor. Add melted chocolate and the rest of the ingredients except for the strawberry topping. Blend until a smooth creamy consistency is achieved. Scrape down sides of bowl as necessary.
3. Spoon the mixture into serving glasses, top with sliced strawberries (or other preferred toppings) and serve as a pudding. To enjoy a mousse-like consistency, refrigerate for at least 2 hours. Can be stored in an airtight container in the refrigerator for up to 7 days.

Spiced Kale Chips

Nutritional Information:
Total fat: 3g
Cholesterol: 0mg
Sodium: 124mg
Total carbohydrates: 1.8g
Dietary fiber: 0.7g
Protein: 0.9g
Calcium: 30mg
Potassium: 100mg
Iron: 0mg
Vitamin D: 0mcg
Time: 30 minutes
Serving Size: 5
Ingredients:
- 1 bunch curly kale
- 1 tbsp olive oil
- ¼ tsp of salt
- ⅛ tsp garlic powder
- ⅛ tsp black pepper

Directions:
1. Preheat the oven to 300 degrees F.
2. Prepare a baking sheet by lining it with aluminum foil.
3. Rinse and dry kale thoroughly by spinning in a salad spinner or patting with paper towels.
4. Tear kale leaves off the stems and break into pieces the size of potato chips. Place into a large mixing bowl and add the rest of the ingredients. Toss so that the kale leaves are thoroughly coated with the spices and oil.
5. Place the coated kale leaves in an even layer that does not overlap on a wire baking rack. Place the wire baking rack atop the foil lined baking sheet.
6. Bake for 20 minutes or until the edges of the kale leaves are crispy.
7. Allow to cool and serve.

Coconut Fat Cups

Nutritional Information:
Total fat: 11.7g
Cholesterol: 0mg
Sodium: 4mg
Total carbohydrates: 2.5g
Dietary fiber: 1.7g
Protein: 0.7g
Calcium: 3mg
Potassium: 10mg
Iron: 1mg
Vitamin D: 0mcg
Time: 1 hour 15 minutes
Serving Size: 10
Ingredients:
- ¼ cup coconut butter, melted
- ¼ cup coconut oil, melted
- 3 drops liquid stevia
- ⅓ cup shredded coconut

Directions:
1. Add all ingredients to a medium mixing bowl and thoroughly combine.
2. Using a tablespoon, fill mini cupcake liners or an ice cube tray with the mixture.
3. Freeze for at least 1 hour and serve. Can be stored in the refrigerator for up to 3 days in an airtight container.

Almond Coconut Fat Cups

Nutritional Information:
Total fat: 4.7g
Cholesterol: 0mg
Sodium: 0mg
Total carbohydrates: 0.9g
Dietary fiber: 0.5g
Protein: 0.4g
Calcium: 4mg
Potassium: 29mg
Iron: 0mg
Vitamin D: 0mcg
Time: 1 hour 10 minutes
Serving Size: 16
Ingredients:
- 3 tbsp almonds, sliced
- 3 tbsp shredded coconut
- 2 tbsp cocoa powder
- ½ tsp almond extract
- ¼ tsp of vanilla extract
- 4 drops liquid stevia
- ¼ cup coconut oil, melted
- ¼ cup coconut butter, melted

Directions:
1. Combine coconut butter, coconut oil, cocoa powder, almond extract, vanilla extract and liquid stevia in a medium mixing bowl.
2. Fold in coconut flakes and sliced almonds.
3. Using a tablespoon, fill mini cupcake liners or an ice cube tray with the mixture.
4. Freeze for at least 1 hour and serve. Can be stored in the refrigerator for up to 3 days in an airtight container.

Candied Toasted Cashew Nuts

Nutritional Information:
Total fat: 3.3g
Cholesterol: 0mg
Sodium: 54mg
Total carbohydrates: 1.6g
Dietary fiber: 0.4g
Protein: 1.2g
Calcium: 3mg
Potassium: 2mg
Iron: 0mg
Vitamin D: 0mcg
Time: 15 minutes
Serving Size: 22

Ingredients:
- 3 cups unsalted cashew nuts
- 1 pack granulated monk fruit sweetener
- 1/2 tsp salt
- 1 tsp vanilla extract
- 1 tbsp cinnamon
- 1/4 cup water

Directions:
1. Place a large skillet over medium heat. When the pan is hot, add monk fruit sweetener, cinnamon, salt, water and vanilla extract. Stir to combine and allow to heat.
2. When the monk fruit sweetener has dissolved, add cashews and stir to ensure that all the cashews are coated with syrup mixture. Continue to stir the cashew mixture until the liquid begins to crystallize on the cashews.
3. Remove the pan from the heat and allow to cool. Stir occasionally to ensure that clusters do not form. Allow the candied cashews to cool completely before serving.

Almond Cookies

Nutritional Information:
Total fat: 1.1g
Cholesterol: 0mg
Sodium: 36mg
Total carbohydrates: 1.7g
Dietary fiber: 0.3g
Protein: 0.5g
Calcium: 19mg
Potassium: 36mg
Iron: 0mg
Vitamin D: 0mcg
Time: 35 minutes
Serving Size: 20
Ingredients:
● 1 cup almond flour
● 1 tbsp flax meal
● 4 tsp granulated erythritol
● ½ tsp almond extract
● ½ cup unsweetened almond milk
● 1 tsp almond extract
● ½ cup almond butter
● ¼ tsp salt
● 1 tsp baking powder
Directions:
1. Preheat your oven to 350 degrees F.
2. Prepare a baking sheet by lining it with parchment paper.
3. Sift almond flour, flax meal, erythritol, baking powder and salt into a large mixing.
4. In another mixing bowl, stir together the rest of the ingredients to form a wet mixture.
5. Fold in wet mixture into the dry ingredients to form a smooth, even batter.
6. Scoop spoonfuls of batter and place onto prepared baking sheet.
7. Flatten slightly and bake for 25 minutes or until cookies are golden brown.
8. Allow to cool then serve.

Coconut Protein Crackers

Nutritional Information:
Total fat: 3.7g
Cholesterol: 0mg
Sodium: 34mg
Total carbohydrates: 1.9g
Dietary fiber: 1.3g
Protein: 1.4g
Calcium: 33mg
Potassium: 22mg
Iron: 1mg
Vitamin D: 0mcg
Time: 1 hour 20 minutes
Serving Size: 20

Ingredients:
- ½ cup unsweetened shredded coconut
- ½ cup vanilla protein powder
- 3 tbsp ground flax seed
- 3 tbsp sesame seed
- 1 tbsp chia seed
- 1 tbsp coconut oil, melted
- ¼ tsp salt
- ½ cup water

Directions:
1. Preheat your oven to 300 degrees F.
2. Prepare a baking sheet by lining it with parchment paper.
3. Prepare egg substitute by combining flax seeds and water in a small bowl. Set aside for 5 minutes.
4. In a large mixing bowl, combine shredded coconut, sesame seeds, chia seeds, salt and protein powder. Mix well.
5. Add coconut oil and flax egg and fold into dry ingredients to incorporate well.
6. Transfer prepared dough onto prepared baking sheet. Spread the mixture as evenly as possible and score to form evenly sized crackers.
7. Bake for 1 hour.
8. Remove baking tray from oven and flip crackers. Place in the oven once more and bake for another 15 minutes.
9. Remove crackers from the oven and allow to cool completely before breaking into individual crackers. Serve.

Raw Strawberry Crumble

Nutritional Information:
Total fat: 15.7g
Cholesterol: 5mg
Sodium: 43mg
Total carbohydrates: 6.1g
Dietary fiber: 3.7g
Protein: 13.1g
Calcium: 216mg
Potassium: 320mg
Iron: 1mg
Vitamin D: 0mcg
Time: 5 minutes
Serving Size: 6
Ingredients:
- 4 cups fresh strawberries, hulled and sliced
- ¼ cup unsweetened coconut flakes
- ½ cup raw walnuts
- ½ tbsp ginger, grated
- ½ tbsp ground cinnamon

Directions:
1. Arrange sliced strawberries on the bottom of a pie dish or serving bowls.
2. Add all of the rest of the ingredients to a food processor and pulse until a crumble consistency is.
3. Arrange the crumble on top of the strawberries and serve.

Peanut Butter Energy Bars

Nutritional Information:
Total fat: 17g
Cholesterol: 0mg
Sodium: 6mg
Total carbohydrates: 13.8g
Dietary fiber: 4.9g
Protein: 9.1g
Calcium: 14mg
Potassium: 209mg
Iron: 1mg
Vitamin D: 0mcg
Time: 10 minutes
Serving Size: 8
Ingredients:
- 1 cup smooth peanut butter
- 4 tsp granulated erythritol
- ⅓ cup coconut flour
- 2 tbsp water

Directions:
1. Prepare a 9-inch loaf pan by lining it with parchment paper.
2. Mix erythritol, peanut butter and water in a medium bowl until a smooth consistency is achieved.
3. Stir in coconut flour and blend well to make a very thick but not dry mixture. If the mixture of appears dry, add a few more teaspoons of water.
4. Press mixture into prepared loaf pan.
5. Refrigerate for at least 2 hours or until set firm.
6. Remove the chilled bars from the loaf pan and cut into bars. Serve. Can be stored in an airtight container in the refrigerator for up to 1 month or in the freezer for up to 6 months.

Lemon Squares

Nutritional Information:
Total fat: 18.1g
Cholesterol: 0mg
Sodium: 2mg
Total carbohydrates: 4.6g
Dietary fiber: 2g
Protein: 1.5g
Calcium: 12mg
Potassium: 57mg
Iron: 0mg
Vitamin D: 0mcg
Time: 5 minutes
Serving Size: 10
Ingredients:
- ¼ cup lemon juice
- ¼ cup coconut oil, melted
- 1 cup unsweetened coconut flakes
- 1 cup macadamia nuts
- 2 tsp granulated erythritol
- 1 tsp vanilla extract

Directions:
1. Prepare a loaf pan by lining it with parchment paper.
2. Add all ingredients to a food processor and pulse for 2 minutes or until a smooth dough forms. It should resemble cookie dough. Scrape down sides of bowl as necessary.
3. Transfer the dough to the prepared baking pan and smooth.
4. Chill in the freezer for 15 minutes or until set.
5. Remove the squares from the loaf pan and slice. Serve. Can be stored in the refrigerator in an airtight container for up to 5 days.

Apple Cider Donuts

Nutritional Information:
Total fat: 17.6g
Cholesterol: 0mg
Sodium: 41mg
Total carbohydrates: 13.3g
Dietary fiber: 8g
Protein: 2.8g
Calcium: 20mg
Potassium: 78mg
Iron: 1mg
Vitamin D: 0mcg
Time: 45 minutes
Serving Size: 6
Ingredients:
- 1 tbsp apple cider vinegar
- 1 tsp vanilla extract
- ½ cup coconut butter
- ½ cup coconut milk
- 1 tbsp granulated erythritol
- 3 tbsp coconut flour
- ¼ tsp baking powder
- ¼ tsp ground cinnamon
- A pinch of salt
- A pinch of nutmeg
- ¼ tbsp psyllium husk

Directions:
1. Preheat your oven to 350 degrees F.
2. Grease a standard donut pan.
3. Combine coconut butter, coconut milk, apple cider vinegar, vanilla extract and erythritol in over a double boiler until the coconut butter is melted and an even, uniform mixture is formed. This will take approximately 5 minutes.
4. Combine the rest of the ingredients into a medium mixing bowl.
5. Pour coconut butter mixture into the dry ingredients. Mix well. Let mixture sit for about 5 minutes.
6. Evenly distribute the batter into 6 of the donut pan cavities. Smooth the top of each donut.
7. Bake for 30 minutes or until edges are golden brown and a toothpick comes how to clean when inserted into the thickest part of the donut.
8. Remove from the oven and allow to cool completely before removing from pan. Serve.

Chapter 9: Smoothies and Other Beverage Recipes

As part of choosing to follow a keto vegan diet, you will realize that most fruits are off limits. Fruits are typically a major ingredient in smoothies, juices and teas. The natural sweetness packs smoothies and juices with delicious flavor while they provide great nutrition in the form of vitamins, minerals and antioxidants.

Unfortunately, fruits are typically naturally high in sugar (carbohydrates). Consuming typical smoothies will kick your body out of ketosis. Therefore, most fruits need to be avoided.

While typical fruit-based smoothies are off limits, you can still indulge in delicious smoothies, juices and sweet teas. All you have to do is change your fruit choices to berries in moderate quantities and change your fruit pieces to vegetable bases. Cauliflower, zucchini and avocado are great fruit substitutes. Add ingredients like vanilla extract, coconut, cinnamon and cocoa and you've got a treat for your taste buds that is also great for your body.

Below you can find recipes for smoothies, juices and warm beverages that your taste buds with love and that will keep your body within ketosis limits.

Matcha Spinach Smoothie

Nutritional Information:
Total fat: 20.8g
Cholesterol: 1mg
Sodium: 19mg
Total carbohydrates: 10.6g
Dietary fiber: 3.6g
Protein: 4g
Calcium: 51mg
Potassium: 312mg
Iron: 1mg
Vitamin D: 0mcg
Time: 5 minutes
Serving Size: 3
Ingredients:
- ½ cup spinach
- ½ tsp matcha powder
- ½ medium avocado
- 1 tbsp MCT oil
- 1 tsp pure vanilla extract
- 1 tbsp granulated erythritol
- ½ cup coconut milk
- ⅔ cup water
- ⅓ cup ice cubes
- ¼ scoop vanilla protein powder

Directions:
1. Add all ingredients to a blender and blend until a smooth consistency is achieved. Serve.

Protein-Packed Blueberry Smoothie

Nutritional Information:
Total fat: 6.1g
Cholesterol: 3mg
Sodium: 73mg
Total carbohydrates: 6g
Dietary fiber: 0.8g
Protein: 6.4g
Calcium: 175mg
Potassium: 79mg
Iron: 1mg
Vitamin D: 0mcg
Time: 5 minutes
Serving Size: 2
Ingredients:
- ¾ unsweetened coconut milk
- ½ cup unsweetened almond milk
- ⅓ cup frozen blueberries
- 4 tbsp vanilla protein powder

Directions:
1. Add all ingredients to a blender and blend until a smooth consistency is achieved. Serve.

Chocolate Avocado Smoothie

Nutritional Information:
Total fat: 18.7g
Cholesterol: 0mg
Sodium: 12mg
Total carbohydrates: 8.1g
Dietary fiber: 4.7g
Protein: 4.3g
Calcium: 10mg
Potassium: 312mg
Iron: 2mg
Vitamin D: 0mcg
Time: 5 minutes
Serving Size: 2
Ingredients:
- 1 tbsp cocoa powder
- ½ medium avocado
- ¾ cup full-fat coconut milk
- ⅓ cup ice cubes
- 1 tbsp natural peanut butter
- 2 drops liquid stevia

Directions:
1. Add all ingredients to a blender and blend until a smooth consistency is achieved. Serve.

Mint Cauliflower Smoothie

Nutritional Information:
Total fat: 19.3g
Cholesterol: 5mg
Sodium: 123mg
Total carbohydrates: 8.8g
Dietary fiber: 5.1g
Protein: 13.7g
Calcium: 223mg
Potassium: 426mg
Iron: 1mg
Vitamin D: 0mcg
Time: 5 minutes
Serving Size: 2
Ingredients:
- ½ cup frozen cauliflower
- 1 tbsp mint, chopped
- ⅓ cup full fat coconut milk
- ⅓ cup ice cubes
- ½ small avocado
- 1 scoop vanilla protein powder
- 1 tbsp cocoa powder
- 1 tbsp coconut oil
- ⅛ tsp ground cinnamon
- A pinch of salt

Directions:
1. Add all ingredients to a blender and blend until a smooth consistency is achieved. Serve.

Strawberry Protein Smoothie

Nutritional Information:
Total fat: 14.2g
Cholesterol: 3mg
Sodium: 23mg
Total carbohydrates: 7.5g
Dietary fiber: 2.4g
Protein: 8.4g
Calcium: 116mg
Potassium: 178mg
Iron: 2mg
Vitamin D: 0mcg
Time: 5 minutes
Serving Size: 2
Ingredients:
- ½ cup frozen strawberries
- 1 tbsp almond butter
- ½ scoop vanilla protein powder
- ⅓ cup almond milk
- ½ cup ice

Directions:
1. Add all ingredients to a blender and blend until a smooth consistency is achieved. Serve.

Turmeric Avocado Smoothie

Nutritional Information:
Total fat: 27.3g
Cholesterol: 0mg
Sodium: 19mg
Total carbohydrates: 10.9g
Dietary fiber: 5g
Protein: 9.6g
Calcium: 65mg
Potassium: 685mg
Iron: 4mg
Vitamin D: 0mcg
Time: 5 minutes
Serving Size: 2
Ingredients:
- ¼ tsp turmeric powder
- 1/2 medium avocado
- 1 cup water
- 1 tbsp MCT oil
- ½ cucumber
- 3 kale leaves
- 2 tbsp of parsley
- 3 tbsp hemp seed
- 1 tbsp lemon juice

Directions:
1. Add all ingredients to a blender and blend until a smooth consistency is achieved. Serve.

Raspberry Avocado Smoothie

Nutritional Information:
Total fat: 19.8g
Cholesterol: 0mg
Sodium: 13mg
Total carbohydrates: 10.8g
Dietary fiber: 7.8g
Protein: 2.2g
Calcium: 21mg
Potassium: 531mg
Iron: 1mg
Vitamin D: 0mcg
Time: 5 minutes
Serving Size: 2
Ingredients:
- 1 small ripe avocado, peeled and pitted
- ¼ cup raspberries, frozen
- 2 tbsp lemon juice
- 1 cup water

Directions:
1. Add all ingredients to a blender and blend until a smooth consistency is achieved. Serve.

Vanilla Coconut Smoothie

Nutritional Information:
Total fat: 15.7g
Cholesterol: 5mg
Sodium: 43mg
Total carbohydrates: 6.1g
Dietary fiber: 3.7g
Protein: 13.1g
Calcium: 216mg
Potassium: 320mg
Iron: 1mg
Vitamin D: 0mcg
Time: 5 minutes
Serving Size: 2
Ingredients:
- 1 scoop vanilla protein powder
- ¼ cup full fat coconut milk
- ½ small avocado
- ½ tbsp of coconut oil, melted
- 1 tbsp sunflower seed
- ½ cup spinach
- ¼ tsp stevia powder
- ½ cup ice cubes

Directions:
8. Add all ingredients to a blender and blend until a smooth consistency is achieved. Serve.

Cleansing Green Spinach Juice

Nutritional Information:
Total fat: 3.7g
Cholesterol: 0mg
Sodium: 226mg
Total carbohydrates: 8.1g
Dietary fiber: 1.7g
Protein: 2.9g
Calcium: 92mg
Potassium: 456mg
Iron: 2mg
Vitamin D: 0mcg
Time: 5 minutes
Serving Size: 2
Ingredients:
- 6 kale leaves
- 2 cups spinach
- 1 inch fresh ginger piece, peeled
- 4 mint leaves
- ½ cucumber, peeled and chopped

Directions:
1. Ensure that vegetable pieces are cut into sizes that will fit into your juicer and juice all ingredients. Serve.

Lime Kale Juice

Nutritional Information:
Total fat: 0.2g
Cholesterol: 0mg
Sodium: 55mg
Total carbohydrates: 6g
Dietary fiber: 1.4g
Protein: 1.2g
Calcium: 54mg
Potassium: 297mg
Iron: 1mg
Vitamin D: 0mcg
Time: 5 minutes
Serving Size: 1
Ingredients:
- ½ tbsp lime juice
- 2 kale leaves
- 1/4 cup spinach
- 3 stalk celery
- ½ inch ginger piece, peeled

Directions:
1. Ensure that vegetable pieces are cut into sizes that will fit into your juicer and juice all ingredients. Serve.

Berry Spinach Juice

Nutritional Information:
Total fat: 0.3g
Cholesterol: 0mg
Sodium: 30mg
Total carbohydrates: 9.5g
Dietary fiber: 2g
Protein: 1.5g
Calcium: 46mg
Potassium: 365mg
Iron: 1mg
Vitamin D: 0mcg
Time: 5 minutes
Serving Size: 2
Ingredients:
- ¼ cup mixed berries, frozen
- ½ cup spinach
- 3 celery stalks
- 1 cucumber, peeled and chopped
- 1 tbsp lime juice

Directions:
1. Ensure that vegetable pieces are cut into sizes that will fit into your juicer and juice all ingredients. Serve.

Keto Vegan Hot Chocolate

Nutritional Information:
Total fat: 15.2g
Cholesterol: 0mg
Sodium: 48mg
Total carbohydrates: 4.8g
Dietary fiber: 2g
Protein: 1.3g
Calcium: 84mg
Potassium: 131mg
Iron: 1mg
Vitamin D: 0mcg
Time: 5 minutes
Serving Size: 2
Ingredients:
- 2 tbsp unsweetened cocoa powder
- ¼ tsp vanilla extract
- ½ tsp granulated erythritol
- ½ cup of hot water
- ½ cup unsweetened almond milk
- 2 tbsp coconut oil

Directions:
1. Add all ingredients to a blender and blend until smooth consistency is achieved. Serve.

Iced Coffee Latte

Nutritional Information:
Total fat: 13.3g
Cholesterol: 0mg
Sodium: 93mg
Total carbohydrates: 1.1g
Dietary fiber: 0.5g
Protein: 0.6g
Calcium: 153mg
Potassium: 126mg
Iron: 0mg
Vitamin D: 1mcg
Time: 15 minutes
Serving Size: 2
Ingredients:
- 1 cup unsweetened almond milk
- 1 tbsp MCT oil
- 2 tsp coconut oil, melted
- ½ cup strong brewed coffee
- ½ tsp vanilla extract
- ½ cup ice cubes

Directions:
1. To make strong brewed coffee, add 4 tablespoon of organic dark roast ground coffee blend and 1 cup or less of water to a small pan and bring to a boil on the stove top over high heat. Strain coffee then place in refrigerator to chill.
2. Once the coffee has cooled, remove from the refrigerator. Add remaining ingredients except for ice and vanilla extract to coffee. Add this mixture to a blender and blend until an extra frothy mixture is achieved.
3. Stir in vanilla extract and pour latte into serving cups. Add ice cubes on top. Pour in extra almond milk if desired and swirl to mix. Serve.

Keto Vegan Eggnog

Nutritional Information:

Total fat: 6.6

Cholesterol: 2mg

Sodium: 142mg

Total carbohydrates: 2.8g

Dietary fiber: 1.3g

Protein: 5.8g

Calcium: 266mg

Potassium: 151mg

Iron: 1mg

Vitamin D: 1mcg

Time: 5 minutes

Serving Size: 5

Ingredients:
- ¼ cup vanilla protein powder
- 3 cups unsweetened almond milk
- 1 tsp ground nutmeg
- 1 tsp vanilla extract
- 1 cup raw salted pecans
- A pinch of cinnamon

Directions:
1. Add all ingredients to a blender and blend until a smooth mixture is achieved.
2. Strain the resulting mixture and chill for at least 30 minutes before serving if a chilled beverage is desired. Can be warmed up on the stove top if a warm beverage is desired.

Creamy Golden Milk

Nutritional Information:

Total fat: 3.1g

Cholesterol: 0mg

Sodium: 8mg

Total carbohydrates: 1.6g

Dietary fiber: 0.4g

Vitamin D: 0mcg

Protein: 0.4g

Calcium: 8mg

Potassium: 33mg

Iron: 1mg

Time: 5 minutes

Serving Size: 1

Ingredients:
- 1 black tea bag
- ½ cup boiling water
- ¼ full fat coconut milk
- ½ tsp turmeric powder
- A pinch of cinnamon
- A pinch of ginger
- ½ tsp stevia powder

Directions:
1. Brew tea by placing tea bag and boiling water into a serving mug. Allow to sit until the tea reaches the desired strength. Remove and discard tea bag.
2. Add the resulting tea and all other ingredients to a blender and blend until a smooth consistency is achieved.
3. Warm in a saucepan over medium heat then serve.

CPSIA information can be obtained
at www.ICGtesting.com
Printed in the USA
LVHW051049160323
741755LV00007B/687

9 781649 844400